A WORLD BANK COUNTRY STUDY

Nutritional Failure in Ecuador

Causes, Consequences, and Solutions

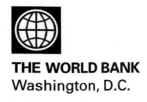

THE WORLD BANK
Washington, D.C.

World Bank Country Studies are among the many reports originally prepared for internal use as part of the continuing analysis by the Bank of the economic and related conditions of its developing member countries and to facilitate its dialogs with the governments. Some of the reports are published in this series with the least possible delay for the use of governments, and the academic, business, financial, and development communities. The manuscript of this paper therefore has not been prepared in accordance with the procedures appropriate to formally-edited texts. Some sources cited in this paper may be informal documents that are not readily available.

ISBN-10: 0-8213-7019-7   ISBN-13: 978-0-8213-7019-3
eISBN: 978-0-8213-7020-9
ISSN: 0253-2123   DOI: 10.1596/978-0-8213-7019-3

Cover Art: "Maternidad" by Maestro Oswaldo Guayasamín.

Library of Congress Cataloging-in-Publication Data has been requested.

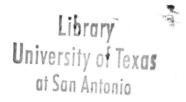

ERRATA

for

Nutritional Failure in Ecuador

Stock Number 17019

ISBN 0-8213-7019-7

On page xxi, in the third complete paragraph, line 2 should say that the PAE "... reaches 1.2 million beneficiaries—31 percent ..."

This Table 9 replaces the one on page 28:

Table 9. Projected Percentage Change in the Stunting Rate Due to Increasing the Proportion of Mothers Able to Recognize a Low-birth-weight Baby

Increase in % with good knowledge:	5%	10%	15%	20%
Urban	−1.90	−3.16	−5.06	−6.96
Rural	−2.26	−3.77	−3.77	−4.91
Poor	−2.92	−5.00	−6.25	−6.67
Non-poor	0.00	−0.66	−1.32	−3.95
0–1,499 m.	−3.33	−4.67	−6.67	−7.33
1,500–2,499 m.	0.00	−5.14	−5.93	−7.91
> 2,499 m.	−0.66	−1.32	−1.99	−3.64
Total	−2.02	−3.54	−4.55	−5.56

Source: World Bank calculation using ENDEMAIN 2004-CEPAR—Ecuador.

On page 80, in Table 35, the Coverage of PAE should be 131%.

On page 107, first paragraph, in the second formula, the *h* should be the greek letter eta (η). The formula therefore should read:

$$N = n(I, Z, \eta).$$

On page 112, in Table C.3, for the 6–11 months parameter, the Large Questionnaire Assets Index value should be −1.11***

Contents

LIST OF TABLES

LIST OF FIGURES

List of Boxes

Acknowledgments

This report was prepared by a team consisting of Ian Walker (Lead Social Protection Specialist, LCSHS, Task Team Leader and co-author), Alessandra Marini (Economist, LCSHS, co-author), Leonardo Lucchetti (JPA, statistical and econometric analysis), Will Waters (consultant, review of sociological and anthropological evidence), Alexandra Lastra (consultant, programmatic and financial review), and James Levinson and Lucy Bassett (consultants, review of international experience).

Piet Buys (consultant) produced the maps. Katiuska King of SIISE (STFS, Ecuador) provided technical support in the analysis of benefit incidence. Nelson Gutierrez and Carmen Tene (consultants) provided support to the study in the World Bank Quito office. Patricia Bernedo (LCSHH) provided invaluable administrative support to the study team at every stage, and especially in the desktop design process. Diane Stamm edited the final version of the manuscript.

Peer Reviewers were Norbert Schady (DECRG), Pedro Olinto (LCSPP), and Meera Shekar (HDNHE). The team received helpful feedback from Helena Ribe, Daniel Cotlear, Keith Hansen, Marcelo Bortman, M. Caridad Araujo, and Omar Arias (all of the World Bank). The report has also benefited from comments and advice provided by Eduardo Argüello Perez (CEPAR), Dan Williams, Gustavo Angeles, and Paul Strupp (MEASURE), Wilma Freire and Manuel Baldeon (Universidad de San Francisco, Quito), Chessa Lutter (PAHO), and Judy McGuire (consultant).

The study team would like to acknowledge the generous cooperation of Ecuador Government officials in STFS, the Ministry of Health, the School Feeding Program (PAE), *Aliméntate Ecuador*, PANN2000, *Operación de Rescate Infantíl* (ORI), SIAN, and INFAA, and officials of UNICEF, PNUD, and WFP in Ecuador.

We would also like to acknowledge the generous cooperation of CEPAR (Ecuador) for sharing with us the ENDEMAIN 2004 dataset; and the generous support of the World Bank–Netherlands Partnership Program (BNPP) Trust Fund in financing the publication costs.

Vice President:	Pamela Cox
Country Director:	Marcelo Giugale
Sector Director:	Evangeline Javier
Sector Managers:	Helena Ribe/Keith Hansen
Task Manager:	Ian Walker

Acronyms and Abbreviations

AE	*Aliméntate Ecuador*
AEPI	*Atención Integral a las Enfermedades de la Primera Infancia*
AINC-C	*Atención Integral a la Ninez-Comunitaria*
BASICS	Basic Support for Institutionalizing Child Survival (USAID-funded program, Honduras)
BDH	Human Development Grant (*Bono de Desarrollo Humano*)
BFHI	Baby Friendly Hospital Institute
BMI	Body Mass Index
CCT	Conditioned Transfer Program
CDC	Centers for Disease Control
CEPAR	*Centro de Estudios de Población y Desarrollo Social*
CESAR	*Centro de Salud Rural* (Honduras)
CEREPS	*Cuenta Especial de Reactivación Productiva y Social, del Desarrollo Científico Tecnológico y de la Estabilización Fiscal* (Special Account for Social and Productive Reactivation (fiscal resources generated from the oil windfall)
DANS	*Diagnóstico de la Situación Alimentaria, Nutricional y de Salud de la Población Menor de Cinco Años*
ENDEMAIN	Demographic and Maternal and Child Health Survey (*Encuesta Demográfica y Materna e Infantil*)
ENEMDU	National Labor Force Survey (*Encuesta Nacional de Empleo*)
FAO	Food and Agriculture Organization
FODI	Children's Development Fund (*Fondo de Desarrollo Infantil*)
GDP	Gross Domestic Product
HAZ	Height-for-Age
IADB	Inter-American Development Bank
ICCIDD	International Council for Control of Iodine Deficiency Disorders
ICT	Science and Technology Insititute (*Insituto de Ciencia y Tecnología*)
IDD	Iodine Deficiency Disorders
IIDES	Institute of Health Development (*Instituto de Investigación para el Desarrollo de la Salud*)
IFPRI	International Food Policy Research Institute
IMCI	Integrated Management of Childhood Illness
INEC	National Insitute of Statistics and Census (*Insituto Nacional de Estadísticas y Censos*)
INNFA	*Instituto Nacional de Niños y Familia*
JUNTOS	"Together"—Peruvian Conditional Cash Transfer
LHS	Left-hand Side
LMG	Free Maternity Law (*Ley de Maternidad Gratuita*)
LSMS	Living Standards Measurement survey
MBS	Social Welfare Ministry (*Ministerio de Bienstar Social*)

MDG	Millenium Development Goals
MEASURE	Monitoring and Evaluation to Assess and Use Results
MECOSUR	*Mercado Común del Sur*
MGRS	Multicentre Growth Reference Study
MIS	Management Information System
MOH	Ministry of Health
MSP	*Ministerio de Salud Pública*
NCHS	National Center for Health Statistics
NGO	Nongovernmental Organizations
ORI	Chile Resource Program *(Operación de Rescate Infantil)*
PAE	School Feeding Program, *(Programa de Alimentación Escolar)*
PAHO	Pan-American Health Organization
PANN	*Programa de Alimentación de Niños y Niñas*
PMA	*Programa Mundial de Alimentos*
PNIAM	Brazil's Breast-feeding Program
PRADEC	*Programa para el Desarrollo Comunitatio (nombre anteriror de Aliméntate Ecuador)*
PRO-AUS	Universal Health Insurance Program
RHS	Right-hand Side
SCOWT	Stunting Combined with Overweight
SELBEN	Social Program's Beneficiaries Database System *(Sistema de Identificación y Selección de Beneficiarios de los Programas Sociales)*
SIAN	*Sistema Integral de Alimentación y Nutrición*
SISVAN	*Sistema de Vigilancia Alimentaria y Nutricional*
SODEM	*Secretaría de Objetivos del Milenio*
STFS	*Sectretaria Técnica del Frente Social*
UNICEF	United Nations Children's Fund
UNIFEM	United Nations Development Fund for Women
UNFPA	United Nations Fund for Population Activities
USAID	United States Agency for International Development
VAD	Vitamin A Deficiency
WAZ	Weight-for-Age
WFP	World Food Programme
WHO	World Health Organization
WHZ	Weight-for-Height

Executive Summary

There is growing international awareness of the importance of early-childhood nutrition to development outcomes. Strong evidence shows that nutritional failure during pregnancy and in the first two years of life leads, ineluctably, to lower human capital endowments, negatively affecting physical strength and cognitive ability in adults. This feeds directly into the reduced earnings potential of individuals and damages national economic growth and competitiveness potential. Faced with this evidence, no country which seeks to be prosperous in the 21st century can afford to neglect the nutritional condition of its children.

There is also abundant evidence that cost-effective options exist for improving nutritional outcomes. In a 2004 review by a panel of leading economists, 4 of the 13 top-ranked development interventions were directly related to malnutrition and hunger, and 6 others were linked to the related issues of primary health and sanitation.

In this setting, the deleterious nutritional situation of Ecuador is a source of great concern. Ecuador forms part of a small group of Latin American countries which report persistently high rates of childhood nutritional deficiency. Like Peru and Guatemala, Ecuador has failed to convert its middle-income status into improved nutritional outcomes. In 2004, Ecuador had a chronic malnutrition (stunting) rate for children under age 5 of 23 percent (almost 300,000 stunted children) and an extreme stunting rate of 6 percent (77,000 extremely stunted children). Ecuador's stunting rate is similar to those reported by several Sub-Saharan countries (Botswana 23 percent, Ghana 26 percent, and South Africa 23 percent).

In 1986, the stunting rate in Ecuador was 34 percent. Since then, there has been a reduction of only 0.6 percentage points a year. If this trend continues, Ecuador will reduce stunting only to 18 percent by 2015—well above the rates already attained by Argentina, Brazil, Chile, and Colombia. To meet its declared goal of halving stunting to 12 percent by 2015, Ecuador needs to triple the historical rate of reduction. This is an ambitious goal, but it is attainable, as other countries have shown. For example, Chile reduced stunting from 24 percent in 1965 to 2 percent in 1980. Between 1980 and 1990, Tanzania reduced the proportion of under-5 children with deficient weight-for-age from 50 percent to 30 percent. And between 1986 and 1995, Thailand cut the incidence of underweight from 23 percent to 15 percent.

The central argument of this study is that the causes of nutritional failure in Ecuador are not immutable, but are the product of policy failure. The primary health and nutrition sectors are poorly articulated and prone to politicization, and they pay little attention to the measurement of outcomes. Ecuador can achieve its goal of reducing stunting to 12 percent by 2015 if it adopts an aggressive strategy to target the relevant populations with the right interventions. The strategy will need a strong accountability framework, with clear goals, which holds the relevant agencies to account based on transparent standards for service production and quality.

Given the structural roots of the problem, the strategy will need to extend to other sectors, such as water and sanitation and education. However, its focus should be in the primary health and nutrition sectors, including the following elements:

- ▦ *Guaranteed access to a full package of primary health services for pregnant mothers and children in the first two years of life*, including: regular check-ups, institutionalized births, vaccinations, growth monitoring, nutritional supplements for mothers and children, and the appropriate treatment of morbidities such as diarrhea and respiratory illnesses.
- ▦ *Community-level growth-promotion in all high-risk areas* is the key intervention likely to make a difference in the short to medium term. It should center on the promotion of appropriate feeding habits, especially, exclusive breast-feeding in the first six months of life, of improved nutritional knowledge among mothers, and adequate complementary feeding practices for children over six months old, together with the promotion of appropriate health care practices.
- ▦ *A more effective national micronutrient program* to improve dietary content through the adoption of international best practices for the fortification of wheat, salt, and sugar with iron, iodine, and essential vitamins.
- ▦ *Universal, computerized monitoring of birth weight and child growth outcomes* should be the anchor of the strategy's accountability system.

The Government has initiated actions to achieve the necessary changes. In 2005, Ecuador established the Integrated System for Feeding and Nutrition Programs (*Sistema Integrado de Alimentación y Nutrición*, SIAN), to strengthen nutritional policies and improve program effectiveness. The Ministry of Health (MoH) has prioritized nutrition-related actions in the country's 198 poorest parishes, and the Human Development Grant (BDH) program is introducing conditions related to the participation in primary health care protocols, which are highly relevant to nutrition outcomes.

The next step is to set clear overall goals and define responsibilities and targets for all the participating programs. They will need to be held accountable through a system of monitoring and impact evaluation. This framework should give rise, in turn, to budgetary assignations that are consistent with the tasks assigned to each program. To support this process, this report provides up-to-date information about nutritional outcomes in Ecuador; summarizes relevant international experience; and reviews the design, targeting, costs, outcomes, and evaluation systems for the existing nutrition-related programs in Ecuador.

A Profile of Malnutrition in Ecuador

Stunting of Children Under 5 is the Main Nutritional Problem in Ecuador. Twenty-three percent of Ecuador's under-5 children—300,000—are stunted, or chronically malnourished, and almost 6 percent—77,000—are severely stunted. Indigenous children account for 20 percent of the stunted children and 28 percent of the severely stunted. Sixty percent of stunted children and 71 percent of severely stunted children live in rural areas. Sixty percent of stunted and 63 percent of extremely stunted children live in the mountain areas (Sierra). Over 70 percent of stunted children live in poor households, as do over 80 percent of severely stunted children.

The Prevalence of Stunting Varies Greatly Among Socioeconomic Groups and by Geographic Location. The stunting rate is higher in rural populations than urban (31 percent compared to 17 percent); higher in the mountain (Sierra) region (32 percent) than on the coast (16 percent) or in Amazonia (23 percent). Stunting is far higher in indigenous children (47 percent stunted and 17 percent severely stunted) than in any other racial group. It is also higher in poor families (28 percent) than in non-poor families (17 percent). In the bottom quintile of income distribution, 30 percent of children are stunted, 9 percent severely so. In the top quintile, only 11 percent are stunted, 2 percent severely.

Like in Other Countries, Almost All Stunting in Ecuador is Produced in the First Two Years of life. Only 3 percent of children under 5 months are stunted. This rises to almost 10 percent in the 6–11-month age group and leaps to 28 percent for children 12–23 months of age; thereafter, it remains stable.

Micronutrient Deficiency. The data on this issue are very old, but very worrisome. The national nutrition survey (DANS 1986) found that 22 percent of children aged 6–59 months were anemic; this rose to 69 percent for children aged 6-12 months and 46 percent for those aged 12–24 months. A recent study reports anemia rates of 44 percent for low-income women of childbearing age. A 1983 survey found goiter prevalence (linked to iodine deficiency) of 37 percent, but since then salt iodization may have improved matters. A 1995 study of parishes in extreme poverty found that 17 percent of children aged 12–36 months suffered from vitamin A deficiency (VAD). Ecuador should carry out a new, nationally representative nutrition survey to update these data.

Causes of Chronic Malnutrition in Ecuador

Econometric Evidence is Presented on the Causes of Malnutrition. An in-depth econometric analysis was undertaken of the causes and correlates of malnutrition, using the rich ENDE-MAIN 2004 household survey data set. The main findings and recommendations are as follows:

■ Children's nutritional states worsen markedly during the first year of life, and then remain stable. *The critical window of opportunity for interventions to prevent stunting in Ecuador is during pregnancy and in the first year of a child's life.*

■ The height of the mother is an important determinant of the child's nutritional status. *Every Ecuadorian girl rescued from stunting now, reduces the likelihood of a future child being born stunted.*

■ The mother's expectation regarding her child's height is highly relevant to stunting outcomes. Other things being equal, women who did not realize that their child was too small at birth are more likely to have a stunted child, today. *Counseling at the community level to improve nutritional knowledge should be a main plank of nutrition strategy.*

■ Children in urban areas have much better growth prospects than rural children. *Nutrition strategy should concentrate on rural communities.*

■ Altitude has a strong, negative association with nutritional status. *Nutrition strategy should give high priority to the isolated communities of the Sierra.*

■ Household's resources are an important determinant, but offer a "long route" to improved nutrition outcomes. Doubling per capita consumption would increase the z-score of the average child by only 0.25 standard deviations. *Other, more direct strategies to improve nutrition are needed to complement income growth.*

▨ Stunting is positively correlated with the number of household members and the number of preschool children in the household. *Adequate birth spacing and reduced family size are relevant strategies for improving nutritional outcomes in Ecuador.*

▨ The availability of toilets has a positive impact on nutritional status. *Investments in rural sanitation are likely to yield positive returns in nutritional status.*

▨ Once the model is fully specified, ethnicity does not appear as a statistically significant factor causing stunting. *The stunting observed in indigenous communities results from their location, socioeconomic exclusion, behavioral factors, and policy failure in overcoming these problems—not from genetics.*

To further illustrate these relationships, this section of the book also presents cross-tabulations of the prevalence of stunting against altitude, ethnicity, and household composition, and includes boxes summarizing the state of global knowledge on the causal linkages of altitude and ethnicity to stunting.

The Double Burden of Disease. Child undernutrition remains Ecuador's greatest nutrition problem. However, child and adult overweight and obesity are also important threats. As elsewhere in Latin America, diet and lifestyles have changed and chronic and degenerative diseases are a growing concern. Nationwide, 40 percent of Ecuadorian mothers are overweight, and the prevalence of obesity is 15 percent. Ecuadorian women are also, on average, short: 14 percent are below the height benchmark of 1.45 meters, normally used to define adult stunting. Almost half of these short women are also overweight, and short mothers are also more likely to have small children. The coexistence of maternal overweight and children's stunting is sometimes known as the "double burden of disease."

Behavioral Roots of Malnutrition. Due to data limitations, this section of the report does not purport to demonstrate causal relationships between behavior and stunting outcomes. Nevertheless, the data are consistent with the international evidence on linkages from health practices and feeding behaviors to nutritional outcomes. In Ecuador, as elsewhere, prenatal and postnatal care, birth institutionalization, weighing at birth, exclusive breast-feeding, the avoidance of diarrhea, and complete immunization are associated with better nutritional outcomes.

Food Expenditure. Stunting in Ecuador is not primarily related to the shortage of food. Although poor households generally spend less on food than the non-poor, within each expenditure quintile, food consumption in the homes of stunted children is very similar to that observed in the homes of non-stunted children. Nor does the proportion of food expenditure in total expenditure vary markedly between the homes of stunted and non-stunted children. However, the share of meat in total consumption is relatively low for households with stunted children at high altitudes, so a shortage of animal protein in the diet may be a cause of stunting in some regions.

Sociological and Anthropological Evidence Suggests that Part of the Problem Can be Traced to the Knowledge, Attitudes, and Practices of indigenous, Afro-, and *mestizo* Ecuadorians toward diet, and illness and its treatment, during pregnancy and early childhood. Ecuador has a rich and complex cultural tapestry, including a significant indigenous (Amerindian) population concentrated in the highlands and in the Amazon lowlands, and an important Afro-Ecuadorian population, descended from slaves, living mainly in coastal areas. There is also a large (mainly rural) population of *mestizo* people, who combine European and indigenous traits. The sociological literature concurs that multiple obstacles exist to the use of formal health services among indigenous and *mestizo* communities, including traditional belief systems, cultural preferences, language barriers, the time and cost required for accessing modern alternatives, and the poor quality of many of the available services. It also documents a generalized distrust of, and reluctance to seek help from, outsiders.

Maternal Diet. There is little evidence of harmful, culturally determined dietary practices during pregnancy. However, there are some practices that contradict modern dietary norms. In some indigenous communities, it is believed that the belly of pregnant women could explode, so it is recommended to drink alcohol instead of water. After birth, lowland kichwa parents engage in fasting and strict control of other behavior, referred to as *sasina*. It is believed that this feeds and strengthens the baby.

Birth Practices. Giving birth at home, often with a traditional birth attendant, remains common among indigenous women. The coverage of prenatal consultation and institutional births is much lower than for the rest of the population. There is abundant evidence that the cultural insensitivity of institutional birthing services causes indigenous women to reject them. Among the lowland kichwa, it is believed that physicians "cut up" women too much. Indigenous women feel uncomfortable with the requirement to disrobe and wait alone in a cold room; it is very important for indigenous people that the family be nearby during childbirth. There is a strong perception that indigenous women are not respected by staff in health facilities. Language is a barrier: very few doctors speak kichwa or any other indigenous language. Women are also concerned that institutional services will not allow them to give birth in the traditional squatting position. Indigenous and Afro-Ecuadorians have a multiplicity of beliefs surrounding the disposal of the placenta, whose non-return is a further disincentive to institutionalized births.

Breast-Feeding. Exclusive breast-feeding is favored by indigenous women, in general, because mothers' milk is free, and is known to be good for the child. There is no evidence that women in Ecuador regard colostrum (the nutritious first milk, given immediately after childbirth) as damaging, as is the case in some parts of Africa.

Management of Diarrhea. Indigenous communities have strongly held beliefs about how sick children should be treated, many of which run directly against the grain of modern best practice. Home treatment of diarrhea usually includes withholding of food and liquids; the intake of liquids is believed to make the condition worse.

Demand for Modern Services. Notwithstanding the traditional beliefs documented above, indigenous Ecuadorians do not reject modern health care per se. Rather, they chose among treatment options depending on the circumstances of the illness, taking account of culturally based perceptions about which illnesses should be treated in institutional settings and which are more appropriate for traditional care, and bearing in mind access conditions for modern services. The interplay between cultural preferences and economic barriers in determining the effective demand for institutional health care is also observed among highland *mestizo* women, who often exhibit acceptance of traditional practices and distrust of outsiders.

Service Hours and Staff Capacity. A critical factor limiting demand for modern services in rural areas and marginal urban neighborhoods is the limited hours of clinic operation and low problem-resolution capacity of the health post, due to poorly qualified staff (such as auxiliary nurses) and a lack of medicines, equipment, and materials.

Policy Implications. These findings underscore the potential importance of the *Ley de Maternidad Gratuita* and the Universal Health Insurance Program (PRO-AUS) in reducing the costs of modern treatment and ensuring the availability of medicines. They also underscore the importance of addressing staffing issues to ensure adequate clinic opening hours, and of improving the cultural sensitivity of childbirth services. Involving traditional midwives is an obvious option. The distrust of outsiders underscores the relevance of training community volunteers to provide nutritional counseling and to counteract damaging superstitions about the management of illness.

Key Issues and Challenges for Ecuador's Nutrition Programs

The scope of the programmatic review covers the primary health network (including the growth-monitoring system, *Sistema de Vigilancia Alimentaria y Nutricional* [SISVAN], and the Free Maternity Law [LMG]); the micronutrient program of the health ministry; the feeding programs, PANN2000 (run by the MoH), *Aliméntate Ecuador* (AE), Chile Resource Program [ORI], and *Instituto Nacional de Niños y Familia* [INNFA] (all supported by the Social Welfare Ministry, [*Ministerio de Bienestar Social*, MBS]), the School Feeding Program (PAE) (run by the Education Ministry); and the cash transfer program, Human Development Grant (BDH) (run by the Social Welfare Ministry).

The Health Network of the Ministry of Public Health (*Ministerio de Salud Pública*, MSP) in Ecuador comprises 1,715 facilities, of which 72 percent are subcenters, the main point of entry of the primary attention network. The system is staffed by some 31,000 professionals—of whom 18 percent are doctors, 11 percent are professional nurses, and 21 percent are auxiliary nurses. Over the last decade, there has been little change in the scope of the network or the number of staff. However, in 2004, following an industrial dispute, doctors' working hours were halved, from eight to four hours per day, implying a significant reduction in the system's capacity. During 2002–04 there was a worrisome reduction in the number of medical consultations, from 861 to 781 per 1,000 population, which might reflect the effect of reduced doctors' working hours.

The *Free Maternity Law* (*Ley de Maternidad Gratuita*, LMG) was passed in 1999 to promote free access to primary health care for mothers and children under 5. The LMG reimburses MSP health centers and hospitals for the cost of services. The LMG's executed budget in 2005 was $19.8 million, about 4 percent of the total budget of the MSP. The LMG has improved the supply of medicines and equipment in the public health system, including nutritional supplements. However, the program has yet to advance significantly with plans to improve the cultural sensitivity of maternity-related services (for example, by allowing the remuneration of traditional midwives who bring their patients to institutional settings for birth). It has also yet to complete the establishment of an adequate Management Information System that allows the tracking of service production and other relevant performance statistics.

The establishment in 2006 of the *PRO-AUS Universal Health Insurance System* will further strengthen the financing of basic health services for the poor in Ecuador. PRO-AUS will be limited to households in SELBEN Quintiles 1 and 2, paying for services not covered by the LMG. However, this also raises the need to coordinate efforts to finance basic health care for low-income families, in order to avoid unnecessary overlaps and fully exploit managerial and administrative synergies.

Growth Monitoring: SISVAN. The MSP's SISVAN system concentrates on the measurement of weight-for-age. Each health post remits statistics for the number of cases measured and the proportion which is underweight, which are processed at the national level. In recent years there has been a worrisome decline in coverage of the SISVAN system. Having risen from 39 percent in 1996 to 74 percent in 1999, the proportion of pregnant women who are measured through SISVAN declined to 33 percent by 2004. Few children are measured more than four times a year, and no mechanisms are in place to follow up on the measurement with effective counseling. Specific children cannot be tracked from month to month, and it is impossible to see what proportion of those measured is gaining weight adequately.

Micronutrient Programs. Until 2003, MSP distributed supplements donated by the United Nations Children's Fund (UNICEF) through health posts. Now, the LMG provides funding for micronutrient supplements, and the food distribution programs such as PANN2000, *Aliméntate Ecuador*, and *Instituto Nacional de Niños y Familia* (INNFA) include nontherapeutic dosages of micronutrients in their powdered food rations. In this context, the role of the micronutrient office of the MSP should be to regulate the provision of supplements by other programs. The second element of micronutrient strategy is the mandatory fortification of mass-consumption foods. In Ecuador, the fortification of wheat flour dates from 1995. The *Instituto de Ciencia y Tecnología* (ICT) in the MSP is responsible for the operation of the system. The iron currently being used (micronized reduced iron powder) provides only about half the bioavailability of ferrous sulphate, which is the preferred form of iron in modern fortification programs. A change of the norm is being considered but no decision has been taken.

Feeding Programs. Ecuador supports half a dozen food distribution programs. These include:

- The School Feeding Program (*Programa de Alimentación Escolar*, PAE) administered through the Education Ministry and aimed at children aged 5 and up.
- Four programs of the Social Welfare Ministry (*Ministerio de Bienestar Social*, MBS): (a) *Aliméntate Ecuador* (formerly PRADEC), which is aimed at children 2 to 5 years of age whose families are in SELBEN Q1 and Q2; it distributes powdered reinforced food, ordinary food rations given as an incentive for mothers to take advantage of available primary health care services, and de-worming pills; (b) *Operación Rescate Infantil* (ORI) supplies three full meals a day to under-5 children in community-based crèches, and pays teams of mothers to care for the children; (c) MBS also transfers funds to the *Instituto Nacional del Niño y la Familia* (INNFA), which supports feeding programs; (d) Children's Development Fund (FODI) (formerly *Nuestros Niños*), an MBS-supported early childhood development program delivered through nongovernmental organizations, some of whose modalities include feeding.

■ PANN2000, administered by the MSP, provides fortified powdered food and drinks (*Mi Papilla* and *Mi Bebida*) to mothers and to children aged 6–24 months who attend public health clinics.

Integrated Food and Nutrition System. Three of the feeding programs (AE, PAE, and PANN2000) are grouped in the Integrated Food and Nutrition System (*Sistema Integrado de Alimentación y Nutrición*, SIAN), which aims to rationalize the programs, to improve targeting, and to articulate feeding interventions with primary health. It is not clear why other programs with similar goals were excluded from SIAN. In early 2006, a new *Food Security Law* was passed. Since this is primary legislation, it supersedes the Executive Decree creating SIAN. The new law has created a new set of mandates around food policy, some of which overlap those originally assigned to SIAN, making it urgent to clarify the role of the latter. The Government should consider making SIAN the focal point for a national nutrition strategy, as an integral part of Ecuador's primary health program, while leaving food policy leadership to the agriculture sector.

SIAN has recently focused on establishing mechanisms to "pass on" individually identified beneficiaries between complementary feeding programs that address different age ranges (AE, PAE, and PANN2000). This should be rethought, since programs focused on children over 2 years of age are unlikely to have much nutritional impact and probably do not belong in the nutrition sector. Rather, SIAN should focus on promoting interventions that are likely to make a difference in stunting outcomes, and should take a lead in addressing the sector's weak internal institutionality. There is a tendency to make politically motivated staff appointments, and frequent leadership changes make it difficult for a clear long-term strategy to coalesce. To overcome this problem, Ecuador needs to develop a corps of technically competent nutrition program managers who are insulated from political interference. Stronger monitoring and impact evaluation activities for nutrition programs, led by the *Secretaria Técnica del Frente Social* (STFS) (as specified in the Executive Decree creating SIAN) would help to catalyze a transformation toward professionally managed programs with clear goals and stable strategies.

Human Development Grant. The Social Welfare Ministry (MBS) also supports the *Bono de Desarrollo Humano* (BDH), a cash transfer program targeted at the poorest 44 percent of families in Ecuador, using a proxy means test (SELBEN). Almost a million mothers are eligible, receiving $15 a month, making this the most costly of Ecuador's nutrition-related programs. The BDH is currently being turned into a Conditioned Transfer Program (CCT), opening up an important opportunity for nutrition strategy. Recent studies in Colombia, Mexico, and Nicaragua have found that CCTs, coupled with appropriate supply-side interventions, can have an important impact on nutrition.

Spending on Nutrition-Related Programs was Just Under 1 Percent of GDP in 2005. Three-quarters of this is due to the BDH. Health spending amounted to a further 1.5 percent of GDP. International comparator data report that Ecuador's health and nutrition spending is about PPP$100 per capita, broadly in line with what would be expected, given the level of Ecuador's gross domestic product.

Budgetary Instability is a Major Source of Inefficiency. Total spending on feeding programs and the BDH has been fairly stable in the last few years, in real terms. However, some programs have faced large fluctuations, and there is also a serious problem of unstable budget flows *within* the fiscal year, due to erratic transfers from the finance ministry, leading to unstable service delivery and undermining transparency. For instance, during 2004–05, PANN2000 more than doubled its executed budget, but the amount it received in transfers was cut by 50 percent. Similarly, PAE doubled its executed budget during 2003–04 and then halved it in 2005.

Cost Per Beneficiary in Feeding Programs Ranges Enormously, from $12 a year for the School Feeding Program, PAE, up to the enormous sum of $534 a year for the Child Rescue Program (*Operación Rescate Infantil,* ORI). This reflects big differences in the benefits, which range from two or three distributions a year of a relatively small value *papilla* (bag of powdered food) by PANN2000 and *Aliméntate Ecuador,* to a monthly cash-equivalent payment of $15 in the case of BDH, and a full regime of three freshly cooked meals a day plus day care all year round, in the case of ORI.

Observable Overhead Margins are Generally at Reasonable Levels, Averaging 12.2 Percent. The notable exception is *Aliméntate Ecuador,* whose very high margin of 23 percent reflects a mismatch between the size of the program's organization and the amount of budget resources it was able to mobilize in 2005. However, part of the overhead of PAE and PANN2000 is buried in education and health ministries' budgets. ORI spends fully a third of the benefit value paying mothers to cook the food and supervise the children.

The Pattern of Program Coverage and Benefits Varies Greatly Across Programs. The School Feeding Program (PAE), reaches 1.3 million beneficiaries—41 percent more than the estimated size of the program's target population of children in rural and urban-marginal schools. But it provides a service for only about a quarter of the 160 days in the school year. Other programs have a relatively high coverage level (for example, *Liméntate Ecuador,* with 69 percent, and PANN2000, with 31 percent), but their benefits are very small and the resulting nutritional impact is questionable. At the other end of the spectrum is ORI, which delivers very large benefits to a small proportion of the target population, raising serious issues of horizontal inequity (other children in similar conditions do not get the same benefit).

Most Ecuadorian Households Receive no Support from Nutrition-Related Programs, While a Significant Minority Receives Support From Multiple Programs. According to household survey data (ENEMDU 2005), 67 percent of households do not benefit from any of the six principal programs reviewed (AE, BDH, INNFA, ORI, PAE, and PANN). Twenty-one percent benefit from one program and 13 percent benefit from more than one. The average annual benefit per household is $109 for beneficiaries of one program, $182 for those with two, $229 for those with three, and $380 for those with four programs.

In an Effort to Fight Politicization and Strengthen Transparency, Many Nutrition-Related Programs Have Adopted Improved Targeting Procedures, But These Need to be Reviewed. Following egregious politicization under the Gutierrez regime, *Aliméntate Ecuador* now uses the SELBEN targeting system (developed for BDH), which identifies the bottom two quintiles of the income distribution (in practice, 44 percent of the population), using a proxy means test. The PRO-AUS Universal Health Insurance System (being introduced in 2006) will use the same system. However, this broad, income-based approach may not be the best way to target nutrition programs. The problem of stunting is more concentrated, affecting 23 percent of children under 5, and is also highly concentrated from a geographic point of view. Because many of the relevant interventions have a community-level focus (rather than a household-level focus), Ecuador should consider adopting a "nutritional poverty map" approach which targets interventions toward the communities where the problem is concentrated (in the rural sierra), and the age range where the problem arises (under 2 years of age). Benefits should not, however, be targeted on individual children with nutritional problems, due to the problem of perverse incentives. A national nutrition survey (as recommended above) could help to calibrate this approach.

Benefit Incidence. The effort to improve income targeting is reflected in the results of a benefit incidence analysis (carried out for this study), which shows that all the programs are progressive, delivering more resources to poor than to rich households. However, there are big variations in the leakage of resources at the top end of the income distribution. In any case, progressive benefit incidence is necessary, but is not sufficient. It is also necessary to get the interventions right, and to ensure wide coverage (small errors of exclusion). This is particularly important when the benefits have a high value, as in the case of ORI.

Recommendations for the Development of a National Nutrition Strategy

The Last Three Years Have Seen Efforts to Improve Programmatic Coordination in the Nutrition Sector, Through the Establishment of SIAN, Under the Aegis of the MoH. Now, SIAN needs to develop a leadership role, which should take in all relevant interventions, including community-level growth promotion, primary health, reproductive health, and population policy (especially, birth spacing), complementary feeding programs, and micronutrient supplementation.

An Important Missing Piece of Ecuador's Nutrition Strategy is Community-Level Counseling, Linked to Growth Monitoring. All the programs currently organized in SIAN are basically food distribution programs, which concentrate on the logistics of the distribution process (normally delegated to the World Food Program [WFP]). In this setting, much energy has been put into arguments about whether to give priority to food distribution for smaller children (PANN2000) or older ones (AE, PAE)-but in addition to getting the age range right, it is also critical to get the intervention right. None of these programs tracks the progress of individual beneficiaries or is concerned, in practice, with the promotion of mothers' nutritional understanding or of appropriate behaviors. International experience suggests that such activities can lead to rapid improvements in child growth outcomes. The BASICS community-based growth promotion program achieved important advances in areas such as Otavalo, but was never adequately institutionalized, so that when United States Agency for International Development (USAID) funding ended, the program evaporated. Ecuador should give priority to establishing a sustainable, community-level counseling system, fully integrated into the primary health network. The STFS' nutrition education project, supported by the European Union, is a step in this direction.

A Sine Qua Non For An Effective National Nutrition Strategy is That it be Anchored in a National Nutrition Monitoring System. The SISVAN growth monitoring system has deteriorated in recent years. It collects out-of-date data for only part of the problem (weight, not height) and for only part of the population (those that turn up at health posts), and then does nothing with them. This needs to be transformed, using computerized techniques. Ecuador should put in place a revamped universal child-growth tracking system, which generates real-time data for the populations of high-risk areas, with measurement sessions taking place in the communities, and not depending on the child visiting a health post.

Because child growth outcomes capture the impact of primary health and nutrition interventions as a whole, the nutrition outcome monitoring system should form an integral part of the national public health network, providing a robust basis for the accountability of health and nutrition programs, nationally and locally. However, since institutionally generated data will inevitably reflect biases (due to the nonrandom causes of exclusion from measurement), this should be complemented by rigorous, survey-based measurement (at least every three years) that allows for accurate inference of the trends in nutritional outcomes.

A key step to effectiveness—as seen in *Atención Integral a la Ninez-Comunitaria* (AIN-C)-type programs—is the sharing of child growth outcome information with mothers at the community level, to engage them in the process of the child's growth monitoring, based on clearly understood standards and goals, and to help them correct the problems that cause stunting. Hand-held computers (used by growth promotion staff) offer a potential technological bridge between high-quality monitoring and effective, real-time counseling for mothers whose children are not growing adequately.

Program Assignment Should be Adjusted, Based on the Severity of Malnutrition.

- In *rural areas of the sierra,* a full package of measures should be implemented, including: community-based growth promotion; improved health service access, nutritional supplements for pregnant mothers and young children, appropriate complementary feeding for children over 6 months of age, water and sanitation investments, conditioned means-tested income transfers, and school feeding.
- In *urban areas,* emphasis should be placed on nutrition education and monitoring activities and means-tested income transfers. Food distribution after 2 years of age should be avoided, due to the danger of producing overweight children.
- *Nationwide,* behavioral change communications programs and a strengthened micronutrient supplementation and fortification program should be implemented.

Transparency and Accountability at the Program Level Should be Given a High Priority. Recent efforts to improve transparency and accountability include new Management Information Systems (MIS) (AE, INNFA, OIR, PAE); more transparent targeting rules (AE, BDH); use of WFP for procurement (AE, PAE, PANN2000); methodologically rigorous impact or effectiveness evaluations (AE, BDH, PANN2000); and modern quality management systems (AE, ORI, PAE). However, not all the programs' impact evaluations meet generally recognized standards for design and quality, and other programs are still working to put their MIS in place (LMG). STFS should assume a stronger support role in the definition and supervision of impact evaluation strategies and monitoring and evaluation systems for the SIAN system.

Role of BDH. The Human Development Grant (BDH) program is, by far, the largest nutrition-relevant program in Ecuador, and should be a central element of the nutrition strategy. The decision to center the BDH on human development outcomes and introduce conditionality opens an opportunity to articulate the program with nutrition goals. BDH could provide an impetus to changes in relevant behavior—such as participation in growth monitoring—which would improve nutritional outcomes. Similarly, the next phase of targeting for BDH (through SELBEN 2) should take account of nutrition issues (not just household income).

Micronutrient Policy. One area where policy needs great strengthening is micronutrients. A critical element of micronutrient strategy is the mandatory fortification of mass-consumption foods. In Ecuador, salt iodization has been implemented since the 1980s, while the fortification of wheat flour dates from 1995. However, the micronized iron currently being used has little beneficiary effect, and the system of control and regulation also needs to be enormously strengthened. Ecuador should consider outsourcing much of this activity to universities.

A second dimension of this issue is the distribution of appropriate micronutrient supplements to targeted populations (such as folic acid to pregnant women). In the past, the micronutrient program of the MoH distributed supplements donated by UNICEF, in tablet form. But the UNICEF donations have ended and LMG is now the source of funding for supplements (both regular and therapeutic dosages) distributed in health posts. The available evidence suggests that this has led to improvements in supply. The fortified food packages (such as those given by AE, INNFA, and PANN2000) also contain a nontherapeutic dosage of micronutrients. In this setting, rather than competing for a distribution role, the MoH's micronutrient program should focus on the regulation, monitoring, and supervision of the provision of micronutrient supplements by other agencies.

CHAPTER 1

Introduction

There is growing awareness of the importance of early-childhood nutrition to development outcomes (World Bank 2006). Strong international evidence shows that nutritional failure during pregnancy and in the first two years of life leads, ineluctably, to lower human capital endowments, negatively affecting physical strength and cognitive ability in adults. This feeds directly into the reduced earnings potential of individuals and damages national economic growth and competitiveness potential in a globalized world. The evidence from Ecuador is consistent with this picture: a recent study shows inferior language skills among children aged 3–6 who are stunted or who have anemia (Paxson and Schady, forthcoming). Faced with this evidence, no country which seeks to be prosperous in the 21st century can afford to neglect the nutritional condition of its children.

There is also ample evidence that cost-effective interventions are available to improve nutritional outcomes. In a 2004 review of the economic returns to alternative development policy strategies, carried out by a respected panel of international development economists, 4 of the 13 top-ranked interventions were directly related to malnutrition and hunger; and 6 others were linked to the related issues of primary health and sanitation (Bhagwati and others 2004).

In this setting, the deleterious nutritional situation of Ecuador is a source of great concern. Ecuador forms part of a small group of Latin American countries (also including Bolivia, Guatemala, Honduras, and Peru) which report persistently high rates of childhood nutritional deficiency. Like Peru and Guatemala, Ecuador has failed to convert its middle-income status into improved nutritional outcomes. Although its per capita income in $PPP terms is a third greater than that of Honduras and Bolivia, Ecuador still has a malnutrition rate very similar to those countries.

In 2004, Ecuador had a chronic malnutrition (stunting) rate for children under 5 of 23.1 percent (some 299,000 stunted children) and an extreme stunting rate of 5.9 percent (77,000 extremely stunted children).[1] Ecuador's stunting rate is similar to those reported by several Sub-Saharan countries (Botswana 23 percent, Ghana 26 percent, and South Africa 23 percent) (World Bank 2006), and the recent rate of reduction has been modest.

Twenty years ago, in 1986, the stunting rate in Ecuador was 34 percent. In the 18 years from 1986–2004, there was an average annual reduction of only 0.6 percentage points. Relative to the initial stunting rate of 34 percent, the compound annual relative rate of reduction was 2.1 percent a year. If the historical trend continues unaltered, Ecuador can expect to reduce under-5 stunting to 18.2 percent (278,000 children) by 2015—well above the rates already attained today by several neighboring countries: Colombia has stunting of 13.5 percent; Argentina, 12.8 percent; Brazil, 10.5 percent and Chile, 1.4 percent. In that case, Ecuador would fall well short of the ambitious goal it has set for itself, to reduce the incidence of hunger by half between 1999 and 2015. To meet this goal, stunting would need to fall to 12 percent (230,000 children, taking account of population growth) by 2015. This would imply almost tripling the historical rate of reduction.

This is an ambitious goal, but it is not unattainable, as other countries have shown. For example, Ecuador's Andean neighbor, Chile, reduced stunting from 23.7 percent in 1965 to 1.9 percent in 1980, a (relative) rate of reduction of 15 percent per year. Between 1980 and 1990, Tanzania reduced the proportion of under-5s with deficient weight-for-age from 50 percent to 30 percent, a rate of reduction of 5 percent. Between 1986 and 1995, Thailand cut the incidence of underweight from 23 percent to 15 percent, a rate of reduction of 4.6 percent.

The central argument of this study is that the causes of poor nutritional outcomes in Ecuador—as in Bolivia, Guatemala, Honduras, and Peru—are not immutable, but are the product of policy failures. The primary health and nutrition sectors have a history of being poorly articulated, prone to politicization, and of paying little attention to the measurement of outcomes. Ecuador can achieve its goal of reducing stunting by half by 2015, if it adopts an aggressive strategy to target the relevant populations with the right interventions. The strategy will need a strong accountability framework, with clear goals, which holds the relevant agencies to account with sector planners, beneficiaries, and donors, based on transparent standards for service production and quality.

Given the structural roots of the problem, the strategy must extend to other sectors, such as water and sanitation and education. Yet, this study recommends that its focus should be in the primary health and nutrition sectors, and should include, as a minimum, the following elements:

■ Guaranteed access to a full package of primary health services for pregnant mothers and children in the first two years of life, including: regular check-ups, institutionalized births, vaccinations, growth monitoring, nutritional supplements, and the appropriate treatment of morbidities such as diarrhea and respiratory illnesses.

---

1. Stunting is defined as having a height-for-age z-score more than 2 standard deviations below the mean for the global reference population; placing the child in the bottom 2.5 percent of the global distribution. Extreme stunting is defined as having a height-for-age z-score more than 3 standard deviations below the mean.

▓ Community-level growth-promotion in all high-risk areas. This is the key intervention likely to make a difference to outcomes in the short to medium term. It should center on the promotion of appropriate feeding habits, especially, exclusive breast-feeding in the first six months of life and of improved nutritional knowledge among mothers and adequate complementary feeding practices for children over 6 months old, together with appropriate health care practices.

▓ An effective national micronutrient program to improve dietary content through the adoption of international best practices for the fortification of wheat, salt, and sugar with iron, iodine, and essential vitamins.

▓ Universal, computerized monitoring of birth weight and child growth outcomes should be the anchor of the strategy's accountability system.

The Government has already initiated actions to achieve the necessary changes. Through an executive decree issued in 2005, Ecuador established the Integrated System for Feeding and Nutrition Programs (*Sistema Integrado de Alimentación y Nutrición*, SIAN), under the leadership of the Ministry of Health (MoH), with a mandate to strengthen nutritional policies and improve program effectiveness. The MoH has prioritized nutrition-related actions in the country's 198 poorest parishes as key goals of Ecuador's primary health strategy, and the Human Development Grant (BDH) program is being reformed to introduce conditionality related to participation in primary health care protocols, which are highly relevant to nutrition outcomes. The next step is to set clear overall goals and define responsibilities and targets for all the participating programs, which will need to be held accountable through a system of monitoring and impact evaluation. This framework should give rise, in turn, to budgetary assignations that are consistent with the tasks assigned to each program.

This report aims to help the Government advance on these fronts by providing consistent, up-to-date information about the nature and scope of the problem (based on both quantitative and qualitative evidence); summarizing relevant international experience; and reviewing the available evidence on program design, targeting, costs, outcomes, and evaluation systems for the existing nutrition and feeding programs in Ecuador.

The rest of this report is organized as follows. Chapter 2 analyzes the scope of nutritional problems in Ecuador, based mainly on a large, national household demographic and health survey carried out in 2004 (the ENDEMAIN survey). Data and maps are presented on the historical trends and on the geographic and socioeconomic distribution of stunting and underweight children in Ecuador. International data comparisons are presented. This chapter shows that the incidence of stunting in children under 5 years of age is concentrated in rural highland areas, and that, in Ecuador as in other countries, the problem is produced in the first two years of life. Data are also presented on other nutritional deficiencies such as the (very high) incidence of anemia, and the (mainly urban) problem of overweight and obesity among children and adult women (linked to the so-called "nutritional transformation").

Chapter 3 explores the available evidence on the causes of the poor outcomes described in Chapter 2, using an internationally recognized framework for understanding malnutrition. The framework highlights three interrelated, proximate causes of nutritional failure in young children: inadequate feeding; low birth weight (reflecting inadequate maternal health and nutrition during pregnancy); and the prevalence of childhood illnesses, which inhibit normal growth, even if a child is well fed. It emphasizes the multiple underlying causes of these problems, at the community and household level, which include: supply-side factors, such as insufficient access to food, to good-quality health services and medicines, and to water and sanitation; and demand-side (or behavioral) factors, such as inadequate dietary practices (including resistance to exclusive breast-feeding and inappropriate complementary feeding), reluctance to participate in institutionalized health care (such as pre-natal clinics, institutionalized births, and child health and growth controls), and inappropriate management of childhood illnesses (such as diarrhea). The second section of the chapter presents econometric evidence on the importance of such factors in Ecuador and estimates the gains in nutritional status that could be expected from improving some of the causal factors identified. The third section summarizes quantitative evidence and what is known from sociological and anthropological studies regarding the knowledge, attitudes, and practices of indigenous, Afro- and *mestizo* Ecuadorians toward diet, and illness and its treatment, during pregnancy and early childhood, and comments on the implications for policy and program design.

Chapter 4 reviews Ecuador's nutrition-related spending and the effectiveness of its programs. It reviews expenditure levels and trends in the sector, showing that, although Ecuador's health and nutrition spending is relatively low in absolute terms, it is broadly in line with what would be expected, given the level of Ecuador's GDP, compared with the rest of Latin America and with similar countries worldwide. The challenge is to turn this spending into better nutrition outcomes through improved effectiveness and targeting (in terms of interventions and of beneficiaries). At present, Ecuador's nutrition status is inferior to that of other countries with similar levels of per capita health and nutrition spending, such as Brazil, Colombia, Jordan, Nicaragua, Thailand, and Venezuela.

The chapter goes on to look at existing programs for primary health, growth monitoring, micronutrient fortification and supplementation, feeding programs, and income support programs. It presents evidence on their conceptualization, planning, targeting (including a benefit incidence analysis), efficiency, effectiveness, accountability, and inter-programmatic coherence. It identifies areas where there is scope for improvement and rationalization and highlights gaps that need to be filled. It also presents examples of successful programs from other countries with potential relevance for Ecuador.

Based on the foregoing elements, Chapter 5 presents the study's recommendations for the development of a national nutrition strategy.

CHAPTER 2

A Profile of Malnutrition in Ecuador

This chapter analyzes the present situation and recent trends in malnutrition (including undernutrition, overweight, and micronutrient deficiency) in Ecuador. It first reviews recent trends for the most important indicator of child malnutrition, deficiency in height-for-age (stunting), comparing the findings of major surveys carried out in 1986, 1998, and 2004. It then provides a detailed analysis of the geographic, demographic, and socioeconomic distribution of different facets of malnutrition in 2004, in order to highlight the areas and groups where public policy needs to be focused to address the problem.

Data Sources

This section is based primarily on the ENDEMAIN 2004 (Demographic and Mother and Child Health Survey), which is the seventh survey in a series dating from 1987 (Ordoñez and others 2005). The survey was carried out by the *Centro de Estudios de Población y Desarrollo Social* (CEPAR), with funding from diverse agencies including: CDC, IADB, Japan, MEASURE, PAHO, UNFPA, UNICEF, UNIFEM, USAID, and WFP. It has a total executed sample of 11,147 women of fertile age, and 12,334 households. The sample design allows inferences to be drawn at the national, urban, rural, regional and (for the first time) provincial level.

The survey collected data on household demographics and epidemiological characteristics, on access to health services, and on knowledge, attitudes, and practices related to reproductive health, on child and maternal mortality, on school attendance, on the use of health services, and on health spending. Going beyond the normal scope of such surveys, the 2004 ENDEMAIN survey also—for the first time—collected anthropometric data (weight and height) for children up to 5 years of age and for their mothers, and on household consumption and expenditure, on participation in Government programs such as the Human Development Grant (BDH), and data on household assets, which provide a basis for relating health and nutrition outcomes to the economic conditions in the household.

The profile also draws on the March 2004 national labor market survey (*Encuesta Nacional de Empleo*, ENEMDU) carried out by the National Institute of Statistics and Censuses (INEC). This quarterly survey provides data on education, migration, employment, and income. For the March 2004 survey—which has a sample of 19,000 homes and 82,000 individuals—additional modules were incorporated on governance and corruption, and on children (including anthropometric measurements for 8,000 children under 5, lost children, disabilities, the quality of parenting, and free-time activities). This provides an opportunity to triangulate with ENDEMAIN regarding anthropometrics and the causes of nutritional outcomes.[2]

Previous ENDEMAIN surveys had not collected anthropometric data. For this reason, historical trends were analyzed by referring to data from a 1986 national nutrition survey (*Diagnóstico de la Situación Alimentaria, Nutricional y de Salud de la Población Ecuatoriana Menor de Cinco Años*, DANS), which had a stratified sample representative of the coast and sierra regions, with a total sample of 7,797 children under 5; and the 1998 Living Standards Measurement survey (LSMS), a nationwide survey with an implemented stratified sample of 5,810 households, representative of the coastal, Sierra, and Amazon regions and which collected anthropometric data on 2,998 children under 5 years of age. Each of these surveys generated observations on the age, height, and weight of the sampled children, which permit the calculation of standardized z-scores, comparable with those generated from the 2004 ENDEMAIN survey.

The Prevalence of Malnutrition in Ecuador

The main nutritional problem in Ecuador is *chronic malnutrition*, that is, deficient height-for-age, or "stunting." Figure 1 shows the distribution for Ecuador of the "z-score" for children under 5 years of age on three standard international indicators of nutritional deficiency: height-for-age (HAZ), weight-for-age (WAZ), and weight-for-height (WHZ), compared in each case with the reference population (the heavy black line).[3]

It can be seen that in Ecuador, the WHZ curve broadly coincides with the normal distribution, but the HAZ curve is shifted markedly to the left. This reflects the fact that 23.2 percent of Ecuadorian children under 5 years of age (299,000 children in all) are

---

2. In December 2005, the ENEMDU survey included questions on knowledge of and/or participation in the main social programs in Ecuador, which provide a basis for undertaking a comprehensive benefit incidence analysis of nutrition-related interventions, presented in Chapter 4.

3. A "z-score" is an age-normalized relative measure of growth, expressed in terms of the number of standard deviations (SDs) by which the child's specific ratio deviates from the mean of the international reference population. For example, a child with a height-for-age z-score of -1 has a height which is one standard deviation below the mean for children of his or her age in months. Children are considered chronically undernourished (stunted) if they have an HAZ more than 2 SDs below the reference mean, and extremely stunted if they are more than 3SDs below the mean.

stunted, that is, they have an HAZ that is more than two standard deviations below the mean for the international reference population. In contrast, in the reference population, only 2.3 percent would be in that tail of the distribution. Even worse, fully 5.9 percent of the population (77,000 children) are *extremely stunted,* that is, their HAZ lies more than three standard deviations below the global population mean. The following sections discuss the level, trends, and distribution of stunt-

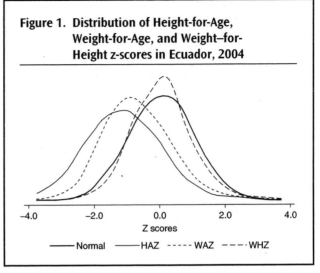

Figure 1. Distribution of Height-for-Age, Weight-for-Age, and Weight–for–Height z-scores in Ecuador, 2004

Source: World Bank calculation using ENDEMAIN 2004.

ing and other indicators of malnutrition—including the alarming incidence of anemia and the growing problem of maternal overweight and obesity.

Recent Trends in Nutritional Outcomes

In spite of the considerable increase in urbanization, improved access to basic services, and increased real incomes following the discovery of oil in the 1970s, Ecuador has experienced a relatively modest improvement in nutritional outcomes over the last 20 years.[4]

In the 18-year interval from 1986 to 2004, stunting fell from 34.0 percent to 23.1 percent. This is an average decline of only 0.6 percentage points a year; in relative terms, the stunting level was falling at a compound rate of 2.1 percent annually. Deficiency in weight-for-age fell from 16.9 percent to 9.3 percent during the same interval. Wasting (deficient weight-for-height) was already almost nonexistent in 1986 and has remained stable since then (1.7 percent) (see Figure 2, Figure 3, and Table 1).

At this rate, Ecuador will fall short of the goal it has set for itself of halving chronic malnutrition (stunting) between 1999 and 2015, which would imply reducing the incidence of stunting in the under-5 population to 12 percent by 2015. At present trends, stunting will still be over 18 percent in that year.

International Comparators for Nutritional Outcomes in Ecuador

The incidence of stunting in Ecuador remains well above that reported by other Latin American countries with similar levels of income, such as El Salvador and Venezuela, and of others

---

4. The ENDEMAIN survey collected anthropometric data for the first time in 2004. However, anthropometric time trends were compiled using data from the 1998 LSMS and from a national nutrition survey carried out in 1986.

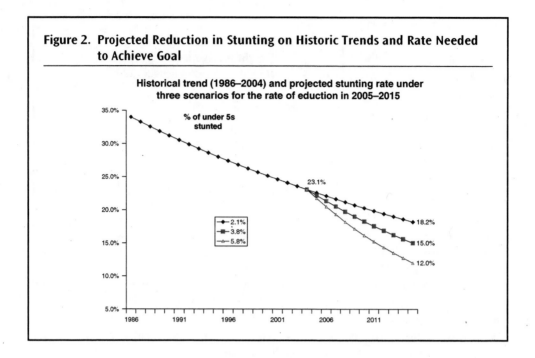

Figure 2. Projected Reduction in Stunting on Historic Trends and Rate Needed to Achieve Goal

Historical trend (1986–2004) and projected stunting rate under three scenarios for the rate of eduction in 2005–2015

with higher incomes, such as Argentina, Brazil, and Chile. The rate is similar to those registered in the neighboring Andean countries of Bolivia and Peru (Table 2 and Figure 4).

Like Peru and Guatemala, Ecuador has failed to convert its middle-income status into improved nutritional outcomes for its population. Although its per capita income in $PPP

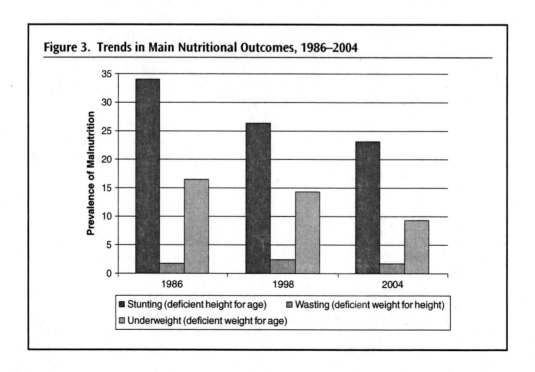

Figure 3. Trends in Main Nutritional Outcomes, 1986–2004

Table 1. Under-5 Nutrition Trends in Ecuador, 1986–2004[a]

	1986	1998	2004
Stunting (deficient height for age)	34.0	26.4	23.1
Wasting (deficient weight for height)	1.7	2.4	1.7
Underweight (deficient weight for age)	16.5	14.3	9.3

[a] Percent of children aged 0–59 months>2 SD below international reference point.

Source: World Bank calculations from ENDEMAIN 2004; National Nutrition Survey DANS (1986); and LSMS (1998).

Table 2. Nutrition Outcomes in Ecuador and Similar Countries

	Ecuador 2004	Peru 2000	Bolivia 2003	Colombia 2000	Argentina 1995/96	Brazil 1996	Chile 2004	El Salvador 2002
Stunting (deficient height for age)	23.2	25.4	26.5	13.5	12.8	10.5	1.4	18.9
Wasting (deficient weight for height)	1.7	0.9	1.3	0.8	3.3	2.3	0.3	1.4

Source: ENDEMAIN 2004.

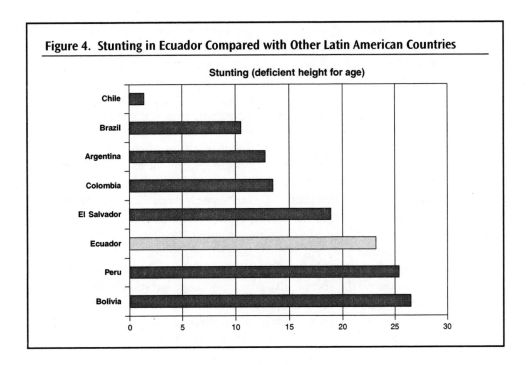

Figure 4. Stunting in Ecuador Compared with Other Latin American Countries

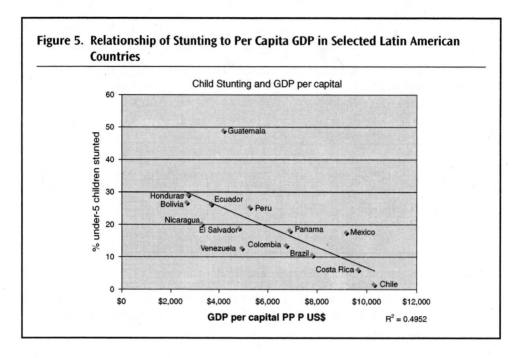

Figure 5. Relationship of Stunting to Per Capita GDP in Selected Latin American Countries

terms—at PPP$3,641—is 40 percent above that of Bolivia and Honduras, Ecuador still has a very similar malnutrition rate to those countries (Figure 5). In contrast, El Salvador, Nicaragua, and Venezuela—which all have income levels similar to Ecuador—have considerably lower levels of stunting.

The Distribution of Malnutrition in Ecuador

Table 3 reports the prevalence of stunting, severe stunting, and other nutritional outcomes within each population group. In total, 23.1 percent of Ecuador's under-5 children are stunted, and within this total, 5.9 percent are severely stunted. In contrast, acute malnutrition (wasting) is almost nonexistent: only 1.7 percent are wasted and 0.4 percent are severely wasted. In relation to their age, 9.3 percent of children are underweight and 1.2 percent are severely underweight. These deficiencies in weight-for-age, in turn, are almost entirely the product of stunting.

Distribution of Stunting. Table 4 reports the distribution of stunted and severely stunted children across the different population groups, showing, in absolute terms, where the problem is concentrated. In all, 298,990 children under 5 in Ecuador are estimated to be stunted, and within that total, 77,095 are severely stunted. Indigenous children (although they comprise only 10 percent of the population) account for 20 percent of the stunted children and 28 percent of the severely stunted. Mestizo children represent, respectively, 72 percent and 5 percent of the total. Sixty percent of stunted children and 71 percent of severely stunted children live in rural areas (although the rural population is only 45 percent of the total). There is also a very high concentration in the mountain areas (Sierra), which account for 60 percent of stunted and 63 percent of extremely stunted children. Seventy-one percent of stunted children live in households classified as poor, and this holds for 81 percent of extremely stunted children.

Table 3. The Prevalence of Under-5 Child Malnutrition in Ecuador

	Stunted	Severely Stunted	Wasted	Severely Wasted	Under-weight	Severely Underweight	Over-weight
Male	24.0	5.8	1.7	0.4	8.8	1.2	2.7
Female	22.1	6.1	1.7	0.4	9.8	1.2	3.7
Age in months							
0–5	3.2	0.1	2.1	0.4	0.7	0.1	5.3
6–11	9.8	2.6	3.0	0.7	6.9	1.1	3.9
12–23	28.4	7.5	4.6	1.2	13.2	2.8	4.1
24–35	24.6	6.5	0.9	0.1	12.3	2.0	1.5
36–47	27.4	8.0	0.0	0.0	9.9	0.5	2.8
48–60	27.9	6.2	0.5	0.1	6.9	0.2	3.1
Indigenous	46.6	16.8	2.8	0.4	15.3	3.5	3.4
Mestizo	21.1	4.9	1.6	0.3	8.7	1.0	3.0
White	18.6	4.7	1.5	0.9	6.2	1.0	5.5
Black	14.2	2.4	1.1	0.7	11.4	0.7	3.0
Urban	16.9	3.1	1.8	0.2	7.7	0.7	3.5
Rural	30.6	9.4	1.6	0.6	11.3	1.9	2.8
Sierra	31.9	8.7	1.4	0.3	10.3	1.0	3.3
Quito	29.9	5.4	1.0	0.0	8.4	0.5	2.8
Urbana	19.5	3.9	1.9	0.1	6.8	0.3	4.2
Rural	38.2	12.1	1.3	0.5	12.6	1.5	3.1
Coast	15.6	3.4	1.8	0.5	8.3	1.1	3.1
Guayaquil	11.7	0.9	1.4	0.7	6.8	0.5	5.1
Urbana	14.8	4.2	2.3	0.1	8.7	1.1	2.5
Rural	20.0	4.9	1.5	0.8	9.1	1.7	2.0
Amazon	22.7	7.4	3.4	0.0	10.3	3.8	2.4
Insular	8.4	2.1	1.1	0.0	10.6	0.0	25.2
Height above sea level							
0–1,499 meters	16.6	3.9	1.9	0.5	8.5	1.4	3.2
1,500–2,499 meters	34.4	9.9	2.4	0.7	11.8	1.1	3.3
>2,499 meters	34.9	9.4	0.9	0.1	10.7	1.1	3.3
Quintile 1	30.0	9.0	2.0	0.5	12.4	2.3	1.8
Quintile 2	24.3	7.0	1.8	0.5	9.0	1.0	2.8
Quintile 3	17.3	3.3	1.3	0.4	7.4	0.6	4.7
Quintile 4	18.7	2.5	0.6	0.0	7.3	0.1	4.3
Quintile 5	11.3	1.9	2.9	0.1	5.2	0.7	4.5
Poor	27.6	8.1	1.9	0.5	10.9	1.8	2.2
Non-poor	16.5	2.8	1.4	0.2	6.9	0.5	4.6
Total	**23.1**	**5.9**	**1.7**	**0.4**	**9.3**	**1.2**	**3.2**

Source: World Bank calculation using ENDEMAIN 2004.

Table 4. Distribution of Stunted and Severely Stunted Under-5s in Ecuador

	Stunted[a]	%	Severely Stunted[b]	%
Male	163,151	55	39,306	51
Female	135,839	45	37,789	49
Indigenous	58,901	20	21,265	28
Mestizo	216,174	72	50,491	65
White	14,833	5	3,784	5
Black	9,082	3	1,555	2
Urban	120,366	40	22,229	29
Rural	178,624	60	54,866	71
Sierra	178,132	60	48,680	63
Quito	34,179	11	6,134	8
Urban	26,571	9	5,267	7
Rural	117,382	39	37,279	48
Coast	102,105	34	22,301	29
Guayaquil	23,919	8	1,785	2
Urban	34,333	11	9,799	13
Rural	43,853	15	10,717	14
Amazonia	18,633	6	6,084	8
Galapagos	120	0	30	0
Poor	212,087	71	62,411	81
Non-poor	86,903	29	14,684	19
Total	**298,990**	**100**	**77,095**	**100**

[a] HAZ >2 S.D.s below the mean.
[b] HAZ >3 S.D.s below the mean.
Source: World Bank calculation using ENDEMAIN (2004).

Prevalence of Stunting. There are very large differences in the prevalence of nutritional outcomes between different socioeconomic groups: by sex, race, urban or rural residence, geographic region, altitude, and income and the poverty level of households.

Gender. The prevalence of stunting is slightly higher among boys than among girls (24 percent compared to 22.1 percent). Extreme stunting rates are very similar for the two groups.

Racial Origin. Indigenous children are much more likely to be stunted (46.6 percent) and severely stunted (16.8 percent) than those of any other racial group. Black children are the least likely to be stunted (14.2 percent). White children are the most likely to be obese (5.5 percent).

Age. As observed in most countries (World Bank 2006:12), the prevalence of stunting in Ecuador increases with the age of the child. Only 3 percent of children under 5 months are stunted, but this rises to almost 10 percent in the 6–11 month age group and leaps to 28 percent for children 12–23 months of age. A similar pattern is observed for extreme stunting, with rates of 0.1 percent, 2.6 percent, and 7.5 percent, respectively, reported for these three age ranges. Thereafter, the level of stunting and extreme stunting remains broadly stable.

These patterns are further illustrated in Figures 7, 8, and 9, which plot the mean z-scores for Ecuadorian children against their age in months. These graphs underline the critical importance of the first two years of life, as the period in which stunting is produced and, therefore, the decisive moment for interventions to prevent it from happening.

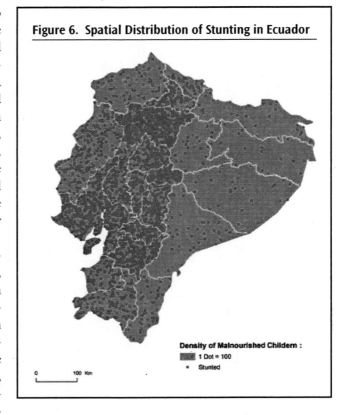

Figure 6. **Spatial Distribution of Stunting in Ecuador**

Density of Malnourished Children :
1 Dot = 100
Stunted

0   100 Km

The average height-for-age z-score (Figure 7) falls dramatically during the first year of life—as does the weight-for-height z-score (Figure 8). From the age of around 20 months,

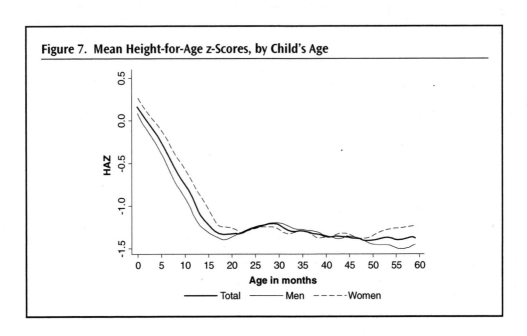

Figure 7. **Mean Height-for-Age z-Scores, by Child's Age**

HAZ

Age in months

—— Total —— Men ---- Women

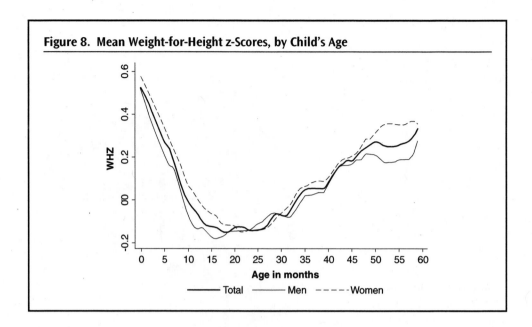

Figure 8. Mean Weight-for-Height z-Scores, by Child's Age

weight begins to recover in relation to height—reflecting the body mass adjusting to the established size of the frame. However, this decline starts from a relatively higher level (an average z-score about 0.5), so that it does not dip far below zero at the bottom of the curve. The weight-for-age score (Figure 9) also improves slowly as a result. However, the loss of stature is never recovered, so that the height-for-age ratio, tracked in the top graph, remains flat and never recovers.

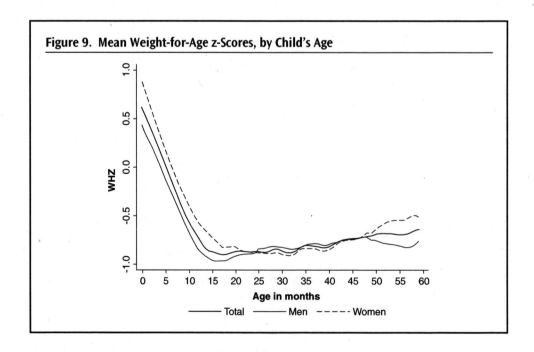

Figure 9. Mean Weight-for-Age z-Scores, by Child's Age

Area. Children living in rural settings are much more likely to be stunted (30.6 percent) or severely stunted (9.4 percent) than those in urban areas (respectively, 16.9 percent and 3.1 percent).

Regions. Ecuador has four major geographic regions: the Pacific lowlands in the west (Coast); the central Andean highlands (Sierra); the eastern lowlands (Amazon); and Galapagos Islands, 600 miles to the west in the Pacific Ocean. These regions have very different rates of malnutrition. Children living in the Sierra, particularly in the rural Sierra and in Quito, have a much higher probability of being stunted (31.9 percent) or severely stunted (8.7 percent) than children in the Costa (15.6 percent

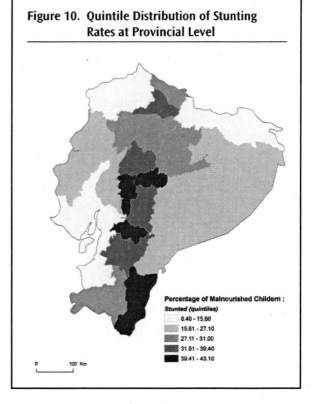

Figure 10. Quintile Distribution of Stunting Rates at Provincial Level

Percentage of Malnourished Childern :
Stunted (quintiles)
- 8.40 - 15.60
- 15.61 - 27.10
- 27.11 - 31.00
- 31.01 - 39.40
- 39.41 - 43.10

and 3.4 percent, respectively). Amazonia lies in between (22.7 percent and 7.4 percent). It is noteworthy that extreme stunting in the Amazon region is very close to that observed in the Sierra.

The regional and provincial differences in stunting outcomes are illustrated in Figure 10 and 11. The provinces located in the Sierra have uniformly high stunting rates compared

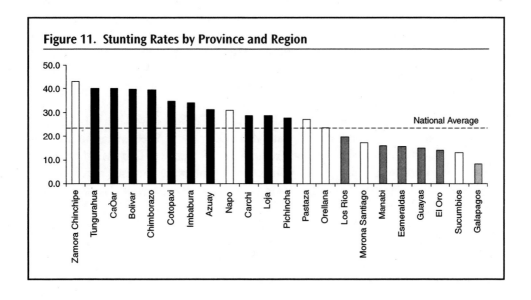

Figure 11. Stunting Rates by Province and Region

with the rest of the country. Five provinces of the Sierra—Bolivar, Cañar, Chimborazo, Chinchipe, Tungurahua, Zamora—have rates above 40 percent. Azuay, Cotopaxi, and Imbabura, also in the Sierra, have rates above 30 percent. The coastal provinces and Galapagos are all below the national mean.

Altitude. Stunting outcomes are strongly correlated with the altitude above sea level at which people live. The critical distinction is between those living below 1,500 meters (where the average stunting rate is 16.6 percent and severe stunting is 4 percent) compared with those at 1,500 meters and higher (35 percent and 10 percent, respectively). The literature on the links between altitude to growth outcomes is discussed in Chapter 3.

Income and Poverty. Income and poverty levels are also correlated to nutritional outcomes. In the bottom quintile of income distribution, 30 percent of children are stunted, 9 percent severely so. In the top quintile, only 11.3 percent are stunted, and 1.9 percent severely so. Similarly, among households classified as poor, stunting levels average 27.6 percent and extreme stunting 8.1 percent; while for non-poor households the figures are 16.15 percent and 2.8 percent, respectively.

The New International Growth Reference Curves

The data reported in the previous subsection refer to the international standard which has been used by the WHO since the 1970s, based on a U.S. reference population from the 1950s. The data presented are therefore comparable with the international literature to date. The normative standard has recently (May 2006) been redefined by the WHO, using an international, breast-fed population reference group. The old reference group was partly formula-fed, a source of distortion, and had other technical problems. Applying the new standard to Ecuador has the effect of increasing the reported stunting rate significantly, to 28.9 percent of the population. This increase is consistent with what has been found on applying the new curves in other countries. The technical motivation for the revision of the international standard is discussed in detail in Appendix A.

The new reference curves were applied to the ENDEMAIN data set in order to see what impact this would have on the reported stunting rate.[5] Figure 12 compares the distribution of the z-scores calculated using the new reference curves with the z-scores calculated using the current reference curves. Based on the new standard, the height-for-age z-score distribution shifts further to the left.

As a result, the incidence of chronic malnutrition in Ecuador is worse than is estimated with the current curves. Overall stunting rates increase by about 6 percentage points, from 23.1 percent to 28.9 percent. On the other hand, the incidence of underweight children decreases by more than 3 percentage points. Both results are consistent with what is observed in other countries. Stunting rates increase some 10 percentage points (to almost

---

5. Calculations are done using WHO Anthro 2005, available for download on the WHO website.

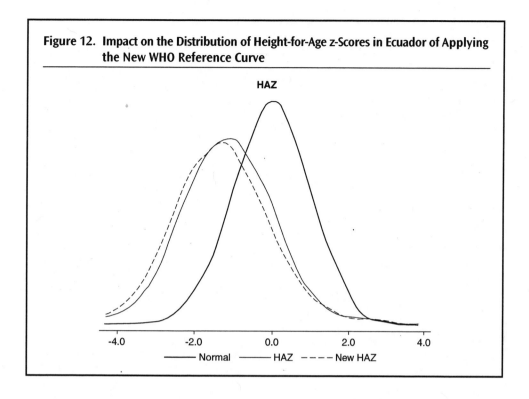

Figure 12. Impact on the Distribution of Height-for-Age z-Scores in Ecuador of Applying the New WHO Reference Curve

55 percent) for indigenous children and about 7 percentage points for poor children, those living in rural areas and in the Sierra region (data tabulated in Appendix A).

Micronutrient Deficiency

Stunting is not the only dimension of malnutrition. Micronutrients (such as vitamin A, iron, and iodine; see Appendix B) are needed by the body for healthy growth and development. Micronutrient deficiency effects health, learning ability, and productivity. It contributes to a vicious circle of underdevelopment and worsening of the conditions of groups that are already disadvantaged.

The study of micronutrient deficiency requires specialized surveys which take blood samples. The last nationally representative study in Ecuador was the 1986 DANS nutrition survey (*Diagnostico de la Situación Alimentaria, Nutricional y de Salud de la Población Ecuatoriana Menor de Cinco Años*). Ecuador should give high priority to organizing a new national nutrition survey to update these data. This section presents an overview of the state of knowledge on the main micronutrient deficiencies, relying mainly on the DANS, but drawing also on evidence from more recent studies of high-risk populations.

Iron Deficiency Anemia. Severe iron deficiency anemia increases the probability of disability and death among women of childbearing age and young children (Mason, Musgrove, and Habicht 2005). Five times more iron is absorbed from meat than from

Table 5. Child Anemia Prevalence (%)

Survey:	DANS	IIDES	BDH
Date:	(1986)	(1993)	(2004)
Sample:	National	High-risk groups	High-risk groups
Age (months):		Percentages	
6–12	69.0	n/a	83.9
12–23	46.0	61.8	76.0
24–35	20.0	40.3	63.4
36–47	13.0	32.0	56.7
48–59	10.0	20.5	47.5
Total	22.0	n/a	n/a

Source: (a) Freire and others (1988); (b) MSP (1995); (c) authors' calculations using data from Araujo (2005).

vegetables, so populations whose diet is poor in meat are more prone to anemia. The problem is often aggravated by blood losses caused by parasites. These factors make it likely that rural populations with low-meat diets and poor sanitary conditions will exhibit high anemia rates.

The available data confirm that anemia is a serious problem in Ecuador. DANS (1986) found that 22 percent of children aged 6–59 months were anemic; this rose alarmingly, to 69 percent for children aged 6–12 months, and to 46 percent for those aged 12–24 months (Freire and others 1988). These are the most recent data at the national level (Table 5).

More recent data for subgroups of the population confirm the continued importance of the anemia problem. A 1993 study of high-risk populations, by the Institute of Health Development (*Instituto de Investigación para el Desarrollo de la Salud,* IIDES) found anemia rates of 62 percent in children aged 12–23 months (MSP 1995). A 2004 survey for the impact evaluation of BDH (whose sample is broadly representative of low-income women and children in the Coastal and Sierra regions) collected data on hemoglobin levels from a sample of 5,000 women aged 15–49 and preschool children. The same survey reported an anemia rate of 61 percent among children aged 0–6 years. For children aged 6–12 months, the rate is almost 84 percent.

Women of childbearing age—especially pregnant women—also have a high risk of anemia. Freire (1989) found anemia of 60 percent in pregnant women attending prenatal controls in the *Maternidad Isidro Ayora hospital.* Yepez found rates of 46 percent for pregnant women in the same hospital (MSP 1995). The BDH 2004 data set reports anemia rates of 44 percent of women of childbearing age, based on altitude-adjusted standards for hemoglobin levels.[6] Higher prevalence of anemia is found in urban areas, in the coastal

---

6. Hemoglobin cutoffs are adjusted for pregnant women, approximately 35 percent of the sample.

Table 6. Correlation of Anemia and Stunting in Low-income Households				
	Mother is		Child is	
	Anemic	Not Anemic	Anemic	Not Anemic
	% of children stunted			
Male	26.7	24.2	29.3	22.3
Female	23.9	22	24.5	21.2
0–5 months	10.1	6.8	10.9	11.5
6–11 months	21.6	16.1	18.6	20.7
12–23 months	33.3	31.5	32.9	31.1
24–35 months	24.6	22.3	25.1	20.4
36–47 months	26.8	21.5	27.6	19.2
48–60 months	23.2	25.6	26.7	22.1
Urban	24.7	25	26.6	23.7
Rural	25.7	22.3	27.2	21
Sierra	27.9	22.4	27.8	21.5
Costa	22.5	24.6	25.8	22.3
Total	25.3	23.1	27.0	21.7

Note: Anemia is defined as having hemoglobin levels less than 12 mg.
Source: World Bank calculation using BDH impact evaluation data set

region, and at lower altitudes. Anemia is also associated with lower education level and economic status. Multivariate analysis highlights the importance of iron loss during pregnancy and the link between higher hemoglobin levels, the quality of health facilities, and availability of iron supplements in the local health facility (Araujo 2005).

Finally, the BDH data set suggests that anemic children are more likely to be stunted. The average stunting rate for anemic children is 27.0 percent, compared with 21.7 percent for nonanemic children (Table 6).

Iodine Deficiency Disorders (IDD). Iodine is needed for the synthesis of the thyroid hormones used in cell replication. Iodine deficiency increases infant mortality, impairs mental capacity, and causes goiter, the enlargement of the thyroid gland. Archeological evidence points to the existence of goiter and endemic cretinism in Ecuador since pre-Columbian times (FAO 2001).

There are no recent national data on IDD prevalence in Ecuador. Subnational data estimates a goiter rate of 10 percent in border regions of neighboring countries (WHO, UNICEF, and ICCIDD 1993). A 1983 survey conducted in 11 provinces found a very high goiter prevalence of 36.5 percent; rates varied dramatically by province, ranging from 12 percent to 54 percent. The prevalence was highest in the Andean highlands, where cretinism was also found. Since the mid-1980s Ecuador has promoted salt iodization. Monitoring in risk areas indicates that IDD decreased significantly during 1985–92 (FAO 2001).

Vitamin A Deficiency (VAD). Vitamin A comes from animal products with high retinol, or from plant products with high beta-carotene.[7] Deficiency causes night blindness and complete blindness. In young children, VAD increases the severity of diarrhea and respiratory infections and contributes to increased mortality rates. The 1986 DANS survey found that 14 percent of Ecuadorian children suffered from VAD, with a higher prevalence in rural areas (Freire and others 1988). A 1995 study, conducted in 534 urban and rural parishes in extreme poverty, found that 17.4 percent of the children aged 12–36 months suffered from VAD; it averaged 22.1 percent in the Sierra, 14.9 percent in the Amazonia, and 12.5 percent in the Costa (ICT/MSP 1999).

---

7. Vitamin A is found in carrots; tomatoes; dark, leafy vegetables; corn; papaya; and oranges; among others.

CHAPTER 3

Causes of Chronic Malnutrition in Ecuador

Chapter 2 described the patterns of nutritional deficiency in Ecuador. This chapter turns to the question: what are the principal causes of these outcomes, and what conclusions can be drawn for policymakers?

The first section starts by laying out an internationally recognized conceptual framework for understanding the causes of child malnutrition. In this context, the findings of statistical and econometric analysis of the causes of malnutrition in Ecuador are presented in the second section. The third section complements this with a discussion of the quantitative and qualitative evidence about behaviors related to mother and child health and diet, especially among Ecuador's indigenous communities.

The Causes of Nutritional Failure

Figure 13 presents a schematic overview of the factors known from international experience to cause stunting. There are three immediate (proximate) causes of an individual child becoming stunted: inadequate food intake, low birth weight, and the incidence and management of childhood disease. These causes are interrelated: disease can reduce food intake, and low food intake increases the vulnerability to disease.

Each of these proximate causes of stunting is rooted in problems at the household level. Low incomes lead to low food intake. Large family sizes and short birth spacing lead to low birth weight, as do poor feeding practices during pregnancy. Poor feeding practices can also lead to inadequate food intake in infants, even in households that do not face economic constraints. Lack of health care (including immunizations) and of access to water and sanitation services lead to an increase in disease. Many of the factors identified at this level of the model are linked to the *behavior* of individuals or families. Reproductive

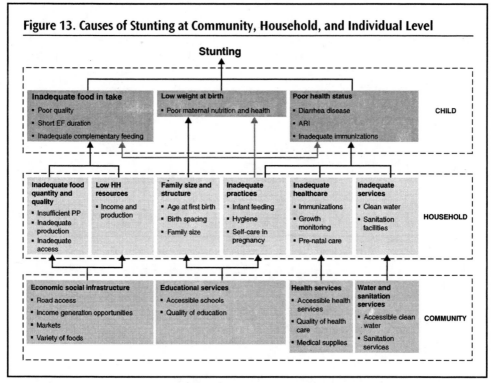

Figure 13. Causes of Stunting at Community, Household, and Individual Level

Note: Adapted from Tufts (2001).

choices, feeding practices, and health care and hygiene practices in the home are all critical determinants of the probability that a child will grow adequately. Each household-level problem, in turn, has its correlates at the community level: the local economy, the education system, the health system, and the water and sanitation system all provide critical inputs into the process of preventing malnutrition. Similarly, underlying the behaviors observed at the household level are the cultural norms prevalent in society.

Statistical Evidence from the ENDEMAIN Survey

Chapter 2 showed evidence of the correlation between stunting and geographic location, poverty, altitude, the child's age, the mother's height, and racial characteristics. This section presents econometric evidence on the importance of these factors as *causes* of stunting.

Multivariate Analysis

The Model and its Results. The methodology for the multivariate regression is described in Appendix C. The model seeks to explain the nutritional status of preschool children (age 0–5). The (continuous) dependent variable used in the analysis is the height-for-age z-score for children aged 0–60 months, an indicator which is directly related to the incidence of chronic malnutrition (stunting).[8]

The model's specification includes individual-, household-, and community-level variables.[9] The variables included in the regression were the following: *Individual characteristics:* the child's age and sex; *Household characteristics:* the sex of the head-of household, the age, years of education and height of the mother, the ethnicity of the mother, the mother's understanding of the nutritional state of the child, per capita consumption, the size of the household, and the number of children under 5 and women over 14 in the household; *Community and location characteristics:* rural or urban area, altitude, and the proportion of families in the community with a dirt floor, a sanitary facility, potable water access, garbage disposal, and availability of TVs, radios, phones, and cell phones.

Four basic regression models were estimated. The first is a "base" model, which includes the basic individual and household determinants of chronic malnutrition. The second model includes, additionally, an innovative variable constructed to reflect the mother's expectations of her child's size (by comparing her opinion of her child's nutritional status at birth with objective data for its birth weight). The third and fourth models also include community-level control variables that summarize the hygienic conditions and access to information of the communities where the children live.[10]

The results of the regressions—which are consistent across the four models—are reported in Table 7. The dependent variable is expressed in standard deviations, so the coefficients of the dummy variables can be interpreted as the standard deviation changes of setting the dummy to one; the coefficient of continuous variables can be interpreted as the standard deviation change in the dependent variable due to a unit change in the regressor (independent variable). For the variables expressed in logarithms, the coefficients can be interpreted as the standard deviation change that is due to the doubling of the independent variable.

The most important findings are the following:

■ Children's nutritional states worsen markedly during the first year of life; and then remain stable. This is consistent with the global literature, and reinforces one of the main conclusions of this study: *the critical window of opportunity for interventions to prevent stunting in Ecuador is during pregnancy and in the first year of a child's life.*

---

8. For the definition of z-scores, see footnote 1 on page 2. The following econometric model describes the causal relation that we estimate: $Nij = \alpha + \beta \chi_{ij} + \varepsilon_{ij}$, where j indexes the household, i indexes the child, N represents the child's nutritional status, Xij is a vector of exogenous community, household, and individual characteristics, α is the constant, and ε_{ij} is a random error term. The reduced form is based on a model of utility maximization over goods and child nutritional status, subject to a budget constraint and a health (nutrition) production function. More details on the underlying economic model are discussed in Appendix C.

9. The choice of variables for inclusion in the estimation was limited to those exogenous variables which are not prone to problems of endogeneity (feedback loops) in the context of a cross-sectional analysis. As appropriate, and where possible (for example, for consumption), instrumental variables were used to avoid this problem.

10. Models 1, 2, and 3 use an instrumental variable approach to the estimation of consumption, while model 4 uses, instead, an un-instrumented asset index. The results of the model remain stable when consumption is included directly, with no instrumentation. These results, together with further details on the econometric methodology, are reported in Appendix C.

Table 7. Parameter Estimates of Reduced Form Models for Height-for-Age Z-score[a]

Model[b]:	(1)	(2)	(3)	(4)
Log of consumption or assets	0.25***	0.26***	0.31***	0.19***
	[0.05]	[0.06]	[0.07]	[0.04]
1 = 6–11 months	−0.58***	−0.58***	−0.58***	−0.60***
	[0.07]	[0.08]	[0.08]	[0.08]
12–23 months	−1.33***	−1.32***	−1.32***	−1.33***
	[0.06]	[0.07]	[0.07]	[0.07]
24–35 months	−1.25***	−1.22***	−1.22***	−1.23***
	[0.06]	[0.07]	[0.07]	[0.07]
36–47 months	−1.40***	−1.37***	−1.38***	−1.39***
	[0.06]	[0.07]	[0.07]	[0.07]
48–59 months	−1.42***	−1.40***	−1.40***	−1.41***
	[0.06]	[0.07]	[0.07]	[0.07]
Male	−0.14***	−0.16***	−0.16***	−0.16***
	[0.03]	[0.03]	[0.04]	[0.03]
HH size	−0.06***	−0.06***	−0.06***	−0.08***
	[0.01]	[0.01]	[0.01]	[0.01]
Number of children <5	−0.04*	−0.06**	−0.06**	−0.07**
	[0.02]	[0.03]	[0.03]	[0.03]
Number of women >14	0.16***	0.16***	0.17***	0.16***
	[0.02]	[0.03]	[0.03]	[0.03]
Men head of HH	0.04	0.01	0.02	0.01
	[0.05]	[0.05]	[0.05]	[0.05]
Mother's age	0.05***	0.07***	0.07***	0.08***
	[0.02]	[0.02]	[0.02]	[0.02]
Mother's age sq.	−0.00***	−0.00***	−0.00***	−0.00***
	[0.00]	[0.00]	[0.00]	[0.00]
Mother's years of education	−0.01	−0.03	−0.03	−0.03
	[0.01]	[0.02]	[0.02]	[0.02]
Mother's years of education sq.	0.00	0.00	0.00	0.00*
	[0.00]	[0.00]	[0.00]	[0.00]
Mother's height in meters	5.37***	5.67***	5.58***	5.60***
	[0.26]	[0.31]	[0.31]	[0.31]
Indigenous	−0.18***	−0.12	−0.11	−0.13
	[0.06]	[0.08]	[0.08]	[0.08]
Urban	0.11***	0.12***	0.18***	0.17***
	[0.04]	[0.04]	[0.05]	[0.05]
Altitude in meters	−0.18***	−0.18***	−0.17***	−0.18***
	[0.01]	[0.02]	[0.02]	[0.02]

Table 7. Parameter Estimates of Reduced Form Models for Height-for-Age
Z-score[a] (*Continued*)

Model[b]:	(1)	(2)	(3)	(4)
Size expectation/knowledge	—	0.24***	0.23***	0.25***
	—	[0.04]	[0.04]	[0.04]
Prop. of families with earth floor	—	—	−0.20	−0.15
	—	—	[0.16]	[0.16]
Prop. of families with toilet	—	—	0.24*	0.20
	—	—	[0.15]	[0.15]
Prop. of fam. w/garbage collection	—	—	−0.17	−0.16
	—	—	[0.14]	[0.14]
Prop. of fam. w/water from river	—	—	0.00	0.03
	—	—	[0.06]	[0.06]
Prop. of families with fix tel.	—	—	0.02	0.04
	—	—	[0.10]	[0.10]
Prop. of families with cellular	—	—	−0.14	−0.09
	—	—	[0.12]	[0.11]
Prop. of families with TV	—	—	−0.34**	−0.37**
	—	—	[0.15]	[0.15]
Prop. of families with radio	—	—	0.10	0.16
	—	—	[0.14]	[0.13]
Constant	−10.29***	−11.10***	−11.19***	−8.86***
	[0.56]	[0.65]	[0.70]	[0.59]
Observations	4,946	3,647	3,645	3651.00
R-squared	0.30	0.29	0.29	0.30

* Significant at 10 percent.
** Significant at 5 percent.
*** Significant at 1 percent.
[a] The dependent variable is expressed in standard deviations. Standard errors are in brackets.
[b] For model specification, see text.

■ The height of the mother is an important determinant of the child's nutritional status-this highlights persistence of nutritional problems across generations. *Every Ecuadorian girl rescued from stunting now, reduces the likelihood of a future child being born stunted.*

■ The mother's expectation regarding her child's height is highly relevant to stunting outcomes in Ecuador. Women who did not realize that their child was too small at birth are more likely to have a stunted child today than those who did realize there was a problem. In contrast, women's formal educational attainment makes no measurable difference.[11] *Counseling at the community level to improve nutritional knowledge and awareness could generate rapid and sustainable improvements in outcomes and should be a main plank of a nutrition strategy.*

▨ Children in urban areas have much better growth prospects than rural children. *Nutrition strategy should aim to "level the playing field" by concentrating on rural communities.*

▨ Altitude has a strong, negative association with children's nutritional status. *Nutrition strategy should give high priority to the isolated communities of the Sierra.*

▨ Household's resources (modeled through per capita consumption or through an asset index) are an important determinant, but offer a "long route" to improved outcomes. Doubling household per capita consumption would increase the z-score of the average child by only 0.25 standard deviations. *Other, more direct strategies to improve nutrition are needed to complement income growth.*

▨ Household composition variables influence children's nutritional status in the expected ways. Children's height is negatively correlated with the total number of household members and the number of preschool children. The number of adult women in the household has instead a positive correlation, suggesting that this increases resources for nurture. *Adequate birth spacing and reduced family size remain highly relevant strategies for improving nutritional outcomes in Ecuador.*

▨ Community-level variables reflecting sanitary conditions (incorporated in models 3 and 4) suggest that—as expected—the availability of toilets and improvements in the quality of the dwelling's floor have a positive impact on child nutritional status, but the coefficients of floor condition are not statistically significant. Perhaps surprisingly, the availability of television is negatively associated with child nutritional status.[12] *Investments in rural sanitation improvements are likely to yield positive returns in nutritional status.*

▨ Once a variable which reflects mothers' expectations for the size of their baby has been incorporated into the model, ethnicity does not appear in the multivariate analysis as a statistically significant factor leading to nutritional failure. We may conclude that the correlation of stunting with race (observed in Chapter 2) reflects factors such as altitude, rural location, income, mother's size, and the tendency of indigenous mothers to have low expectations for their child's size (thus failing to act to promote better growth). The difference between the results of the first and second model suggests that the size expectations variable captures the effect of cultural beliefs and practices associated with being indigenous. *The high level of stunting observed in indigenous communities in Chapter 2 results from factors such as their location, socioeconomic exclusion, behavioral factors, and policy failure in overcoming these factors-not from genetics.*

---

11. Larrea (2004) also found little impact on children's nutritional status from the mother's basic education, but found a positive effect for higher levels of education. The present study found a similar effect in other variants of the model, reported in Appendix C. This differs from results found for other Andean countries, which typically show decreasing returns (a bigger impact of primary education than later levels). Larrea suggests that this results from the poor quality of basic education. He also finds that improvements in maternal higher education benefit mainly the richer deciles of the population.

12. This is not as strange as it may sound. A recent study of urban children in the Boston area found a strong correlation between watching television and worsening in the quality of the diet caused by the fact that children who watch more television eat more of the "junk foods" it advertises (Wiecha and others 2006).

Table 8: Reduction in the Stunting Rate (%) Expected to Result from Increased Consumption

	Growth			Implicit tax		
	3%	5%	8%	10%	20%	30%
Urban	−0.63	−1.90	−1.90	−0.63	−0.63	−1.90
Rural	−1.13	−1.13	−3.02	−1.51	−3.40	−4.15
Poor	−0.83	−0.83	−2.08	−1.67	−4.17	−5.42
Non-poor	−0.66	−1.97	−3.29	0.66	1.32	1.32
0–1,499 m.	−0.67	−0.67	−0.67	−1.33	−3.33	−4.67
1,500–2,499 m.	0.00	−3.16	−3.16	1.19	1.19	1.19
> 2,499 m.	−1.66	−1.99	−4.64	−1.66	−1.66	−1.99
Total	**−1.01**	**−1.01**	**−2.53**	**−1.01**	**−2.02**	**−3.03**

Note: Simulations are based on the estimations from model (4) in Table 7. See text for explanation of methodology.
Source: World Bank calculation using ENDEMAIN 2004-CEPAR—Ecuador.

Estimated Impact of Increased Consumption and Improved Nutritional Knowledge. In this section, we use the model from column three in Table 7 to predict the decline in chronic malnutrition that can be expected from increased consumption and from improved maternal nutritional knowledge (as reflected in their expectations for their child's size).

Table 8 illustrates the potential impact of increased per capita consumption. It models two possible channels through which consumption could increase:

- Income growth that increases per capita consumption across the board by (a) 3 percent, (b) 5 percent, or (c) 8 percent.
- A proportional income tax of (a) 10 percent, (b) 20 percent, and (c) 30 percent, whose revenues are equally distributed among the population (thus redistributing a fixed amount of national income from richer to poorer households).

The results show that growth in income of either 3 percent or 5 percent would generate similar levels of reduction in malnutrition (about 1 percent in each case), and have a very limited impact on the most vulnerable segments of the population. An 8 percent income growth would generate a reduction in malnutrition of about 2.5 percent, which is equivalent to 0.6 percentage points. Under this scenario, the overall malnutrition rate would decrease from 23.1 percent to 22.5 percent. A 30 percent implicit tax leads to a 3 percent reduction in the overall malnutrition rate, equivalent to 1.3 percentage points. The implicit tax has a stronger impact on children of poor and rural families while the income transfer benefits the urban and non-poor population more.[13]

The study found that 20 percent of mothers were not aware that their child's birth weight was inadequate—making them unlikely to try to do anything about it. The econometric analysis reported in Table 7 suggests that their children are more likely to be stunted

---

13. Consumption increases have other benefits, in addition to their possible impact on nutritional status.

Table 9. Projected Percentage Change in the Stunting Rate Due to Increasing the Proportion of Mothers Able to Recognize a Low-birth-weight Baby

Increase in % with good knowledge:	5%	10%	15%	20%
Urban	21.90	23.16	25.06	26.96
Rural	22.26	23.77	23.77	24.91
Poor	22.92	25.00	26.25	26.67
Non-poor	0.00	20.66	21.32	23.95
0–1,499 m.	23.33	24.67	26.67	27.33
1,500–2,499 m.	0.00	25.14	25.93	27.91
> 2,499 m.	20.66	21.32	21.99	23.64
Total	22.02	23.54	24.55	25.56

Source: World Bank calculation using ENDEMAIN 2004-CEPAR—Ecuador.

today as a result. Based on these relationships, Table 9 models the expected impact on the prevalence of stunting of an increase in the proportion of women who are able to make an accurate assessment of their child's nutritional status at birth. It simulates the impact of improving the knowledge of 5 percent of the population (starting from the poorest), and that of 10, 15, and 20 percent. The estimated impact varies from a 2 percent to a 5.6 percent reduction in the overall malnutrition rate. The reduction is particularly marked for the poor, urban population and for children living at middle altitude (1,500–2,500 meters). These results suggest that improving the nutritional knowledge of 5 percent of mothers could reduce malnutrition as much as an 8 percent increase in consumption or a redistributive consumption tax of 30 percent—but is a faster, cheaper option.

Altitude and Stunting

The econometric evidence presented above showed the high significance of altitude for stunting outcomes. It is relatively unusual to have precise data for the height above sea level for each censal segment observed in household survey data sets, as was the case for this study. Figure 14 shows the steady decline in the height-for-age z-score of under-5 children as altitude increases. The impact on stunting is particularly marked above 1,500 meters, and is uniform across racial groups and socioeconomic categories (Table 10). However, it remains important to understand the way in which altitude feeds into nutritional outcomes: to what extent is it through hypoxia (or other similar physiological mechanisms), and to what extent is it through diet and isolation? The design of appropriate policies depends on the answer to this question.

The extensive international literature (reviewed in Box 1) suggests that—although there are important physiological links—the main channels from altitude to growth run through agriculture and isolation, which, in turn, affect diet and access to health services. If so, policies to improve diet and increase access are likely to make an important difference in stunting in high-altitude communities. The quantitative findings of this study on the

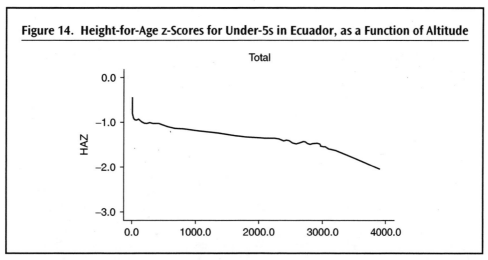

Figure 14. Height-for-Age z-Scores for Under-5s in Ecuador, as a Function of Altitude

Source: World Bank calculation using ENDEMAIN 2004.

links between diet and stunting are presented in the next major section, as are the qualitative evidence on this point.

Ethnicity and Stunting

In spite of the strong correlation between stunting and ethnicity (based on self-definition) reported in Chapter 2, the multivariate analysis undertaken for this study indicates that, once the model is fully specified, (including altitude, the mothers' height, mothers nutritional knowledge, rural or urban location, and consumption), ethnicity, as such, does not appear to be a significant cause of stunting.

Table 10. **Proportion of Stunted Children by Mother's Ethnicity and Segment's Altitude**

	0–1,499 m.	1,500–2,499 m.	>2,499 meters.
Indigenous	26.8	57.1	54.6
Mestizo	16.9	31.4	29.0
White	12.2	31.3	35.4
Black	10.7	29.5	36.3
Q1	22.8	44.9	45.2
Q2	17.7	32.0	40.0
Q3	10.0	27.0	32.0
Q4	10.9	22.0	30.0
Q5	7.0	22.3	14.8
Total	**16.6**	**34.4**	**34.9**

Source: World Bank calculation using ENDEMAIN 2004.

Box 1: The Linkages of Altitude to Stunting

The multivariate analysis presented in this study finds that height above sea level is a strong determinant of stunting in Ecuador. This is in line with international experience. The key question is whether poor nutritional outcomes at high altitude are explained primarily by the physiological effects of height (such as hypoxia) or by the socioeconomic conditions of high-altitude populations (that is, isolation, poor hygiene and sanitation, poor access to services, and limited agricultural potential).

Physiological Effects

Several researchers have noted that early childhood growth is inherently slower at extremely high altitudes (above 4,000 meters) (Haas 1982; Greksa 1986; Obert 1994 as cited in a World Bank 2002). But others claim that growth is similar at high and low altitude (Pawson 1977), or actually more rapid at high altitude (Clegg and others 1972 as cited in Pawson 2001; Huijbers and others 1996). In addition to the effect of hypoxia, exposure to high altitude may also affect child growth through extreme temperatures, high solar radiation, lower barometric pressure, oxygen concentration, and humidity. In the presence of these factors, normal child growth requires increased basal metabolism and higher iron and energy intake (Morales, Aguilar, and Calzadilla 2005; Pawson and others 2001). The "barrel-shaped" chest morphology of some high-altitude populations is thought to be an adaptive response to hypoxia among nutritionally stunted individuals (Frisancho and Baker 1970; Mueller and others 1978; Stinson 1980; Greska 1986a).

There is strong evidence that birth weight, generally an important determinant of child growth, is physiologically affected by altitude. In Bolivia, lower birth weights were found at high altitude, even after controlling for maternal nutritional status (Guissani and others 2001). But there is evidence from Tibet that people with prolonged high-altitude resident ancestry experience less reduction in birth weight (Zamudio and others 1993; Haas and others 1980). In any case, low birth weight explains only a small proportion of overall under-2 stunting, and does not explain inadequate infant weight gain. If properly cared for (for example, exclusively breast-fed), low-birth-weight infants often experience catch-up growth immediately after birth (World Bank Bolivia Report 2002).

Data for children from countries with varying altitudes indicate that while low iron intakes are more prevalent at high altitudes, anemia, per se, is not. This is consistent with our findings for Ecuador, where higher anemia rates are higher in the lowlands. The absence of contributory parasitic infection at high altitudes is a partial explanation. Women at high altitude have been found to have lower body iron stores, but hemoglobin levels in Tibetan and Bolivian studies appeared to relate more to genetic characteristics than altitude. In a 2005 study in Bolivia (Cook and others 2005), body iron stores of women living above 3,000 meters were found to be one-third lower than for women living at lower altitudes. An adult 60- kilogram woman living at 3,500 meters was found to require 355 milligrams more iron (or 5.9 mg/kg) than a low-altitude woman to increase hemoglobin by 26 g/L.

Social/Behavioral Effects

Many studies consider that hypoxia and other physiological effects play a secondary role in the stunting of high-altitude populations. They argue that the main determinants are diet and infection, affected by socioeconomic status and by limited access to health services, education, and markets, all related to geographic isolation (Berti and others 1998; Harris and others 2001; Leonard and others 2003). Agricultures at high altitudes are often associated with poorer crop production (Morales, Aguilar, and Calzadila 2005; Leonard and others 2003), lower nutritional value of food (Leonard and others 2003; Marini 2006), and fewer income-generating options (Morales 2005). As a result, children at high altitude may experience a relatively low intake of animal foods (Berti, Leonard, and Berti 1998; Leonard and others 2000; Rogers and others 2002; Marini and Gragnolati 2006), less access to micronutrient-rich foods (Berti 1998; Rogers and others 2002), and poorer-quality complementary foods (Leonard and others 2000).

This finding is consistent with the cross-country comparisons, which do not suggest a strong link between stunting and the size of indigenous populations in Latin America. Ecuador's stunting rate is similar to that of other countries with much larger indigenous populations, such as Bolivia and Peru (Figure 16), and much higher than that of countries with similar indiginous populations shares (Chile, El Salvador, and Mexico).

It is also consistent with the findings of a large body of international literature which has concluded that stunting in children under age 5 in indigenous populations is not genetically predetermined (Box 2).

This study concludes that the reasons for the nutritional failure of Ecuador's indigenous population are not intrinsic or genetic. Rather, they are linked to the socioeconomic characteristics of the indigenous

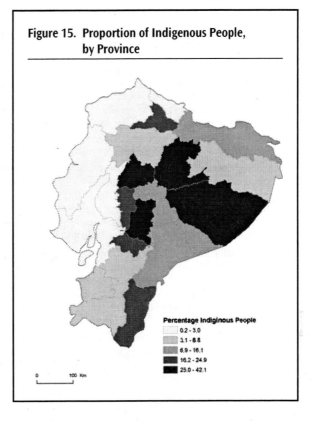

Figure 15. Proportion of Indigenous People, by Province

Percentage Indigenous People

0.2 - 3.0
3.1 - 6.8
6.9 - 16.1
16.2 - 24.9
25.0 - 42.1

0   100 Km

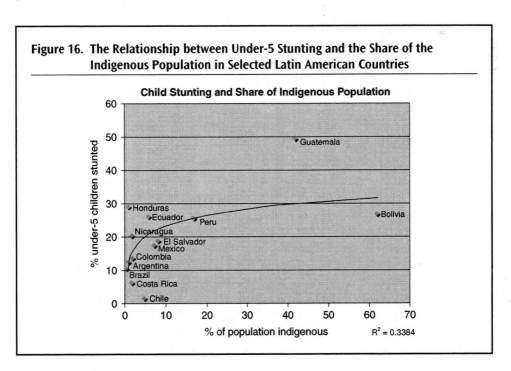

Figure 16. The Relationship between Under-5 Stunting and the Share of the Indigenous Population in Selected Latin American Countries

Child Stunting and Share of Indigenous Population

% under-5 children stunted

% of population indigenous $R^2 = 0.3384$

Box 2: International Evidence on the Growth Potential of Indigenous Children

---

Indigenous populations and ethnic minorities are often disproportionately affected by chronic childhood malnutrition. This is the case in Latin America (particularly in Bolivia, Brazil, Guatemala, Mexico, and Peru), among Scheduled Tribes in India, and in South Africa. It is sometimes thought that this is the result of comparing them with the wrong reference population. The current Centers for Disease Control (CDC) growth curves (the standard point of reference for monitoring growth outcomes) are based on studies undertaken in the United States in the 1950s, of children of European ancestry. If indigenous children had intrinsically lower growth potential than the reference population, this approach would report higher stunting rates for those groups.

However, evidence from numerous studies indicates that indigenous children are not genetically programmed to be short. Although there are clear differences between adults of different ethnicities, children have the potential to achieve similar levels of growth in the few years of life. Variation in under-5 stunting levels is more likely driven by socioeconomic status, social and political exclusion, geographic isolation, and cultural practices, especially those related to maternal and child health and feeding practices (Frongillo and Hanson 1995; Habicht 1974).

Data from India (Rao and Sastry 1977) and Guatemala (Johnston, Borden, and MacVean 1973) suggest that ethnic differences in growth potential are minor prior to puberty, when the main size differentiation among ethnic groups materializes. Research shows that clear differences emerge during adolescence for both sexes: Guatemalan and Indian children who were near the 50th percentile of the reference growth charts prior to puberty, ended up near the 25th percentile by the end of adolescence.

Previous studies (Eveleth and Tanner 1976, 1990) reveal that, on a worldwide scale, height differences among children under age 5 year from different countries are relatively small in comparison with large differences between and within countries due to environmental factors. Similarly, Martorell (1985), using samples of height measurements of 7-year-old boys from Brazil, Costa Rica, Guatemala, Haiti, Hong Kong, India, Jamaica, and Nigeria, shows that, while the differences due to social class were large, the differences that could be attributed to genetic factors were small. Looking at growth data from well-to-do preschool children of different ethnic groups, Habicht and others (1974) reach the same conclusion. More recently, Bustos and others (2001) show that higher stunting levels among the indigenous Mapuche children in Chile should be interpreted as reflective of their poverty, and that the reference to assess their growth is appropriate. The one group that does appear to be shorter than the rest is East Asian children. Children of Japanese or Chinese origin, whether growing up in California, Hawaii, or in Taiwan, Hong Kong, or Japan, have mean height values at 7 years of age that fall near the 25th percentile of the WHO/NCHS/CDC reference charts (Martorell and Habicht 1986).

---

population. As discussed above, there are intergeneration transmission mechanisms, from maternal stunting and obesity to the stunting of the next generation of children, whose importance is confirmed by the multivariate analysis, and which may constrain the rate of change. Nevertheless, many of the causes of stunting in Ecuador's indigenous children are clearly tractable, in the short term, to appropriate policy interventions.

To improve nutritional outcomes in indigenous populations of Ecuador, it is necessary to improve their diet, to improve nutrition and health knowledge, to change feeding and health-care behaviors, and to improve effective access to good-quality, affordable, and culturally sensitive basic health services. The next major section reviews sociological and anthropological evidence which identifies behavioral factors that may contribute to indigenous malnutrition in Ecuador, and identifies ways in which the cultural insensitivity of the formal health care system itself reinforces low indigenous demand, by imposing norms and standards which are unnecessarily inimical to the traditions and beliefs of these communities.

Table 11. The Correlation between Household Composition and Nutritional Outcomes

			(% of under-5s in each nutritional category)				
	Stunted	**Severely Stunted**	**Wasted**	**Severely Wasted**	**Under-weight**	**Severely Under-weight**	**Obese**
Number of Children aged under 5 in the household							
One	19.5	4.2	1.5	0.1	7.8	0.7	4.2
Two	26.3	7.4	1.7	0.5	10.4	1.7	2.2
Three	27.6	8.8	2.6	1.3	12.1	1.8	2.3
Number of women aged over 14 in the household							
One	24.0	6.1	1.4	0.4	9.1	1.1	3.2
Two	21.3	6.1	1.7	0.2	10.9	1.7	4.0
Three	21.6	4.8	3.1	0.8	7.6	1.3	1.8
Gender of head of household							
Man	22.9	6.1	1.8	0.4	9.4	1.2	3.2
Woman	24.4	4.6	1.2	0.1	8.8	1.5	3.0
Total	23.1	5.9	1.7	0.4	9.3	1.2	3.2

Note: Children <5. Stunted includes Severely Stunted, Wasted includes Severely Wasted, and Underweight includes Severely Underweight.
Source: World Bank calculation using ENDEMAIN 2004.

These findings should contribute to a discussion of ways to reform the relevant norms, without undermining the quality of services.

Household Size and Composition

The multivariate analysis confirmed the importance of household size and composition as a factor determining nutritional outcomes. These relationships are further described in Table 11. Higher numbers of children tend to generate pressure for resources, care, and attention. They are also associated with shorter spacing of births, which-as other studies have shown-has a negative impact on birth weight, in turn an important factor causing stunting. An increase in the number of adult women in the household tends to improve nutritional outcomes, probably due to an increase in resources available for caring. The gender of the household head has no discernible impact.

Mothers' Nutritional Status and the "Double Burden of Disease"

Child undernutrition remains Ecuador's greatest nutrition problem. However, child and adult overweight and obesity are also important threats.[14] As elsewhere in Latin America, diet and lifestyles have changed and chronic and degenerative diseases are a growing concern.

---

14. A recent study by Manuel Baldeon of the *Universidad de San Francisco* of Quito found that 100 percent of a small sample of 30 women in the Central market of Quito were either overweight or obese.

Overweight and obesity are associated with an increased prevalence of hypertension, blood lipid concentration, diabetes mellitus,[15] and ischemic heart disease (Solomon and Manson 1997). Studies have shown an association between excess weight and endometrial cancer and between high adult Body Mass Indexes (BMIs) and mortality rates (Stevens and others 1998).

The 2004 ENDEMAIN survey collected data on mothers' and children's weight that allows analysis of the overweight problem in Ecuador. It also permits analysis of the relationship between maternal overweight and child undernourishment.[16] As reported above, overweight is not a serious problem among preschool children, averaging only about 3 percent. However, in contrast, there is evidence of a high prevalence of overweight and obesity among mothers. There is also evidence that a significant minority of women are both stunted and overweight, and of a possible feedback loop to the stunting of their children.

Mothers' Nutritional Status. Nationwide, 40.4 percent of Ecuadorian mothers are overweight, and the prevalence of obesity is 14.6 percent (Table 12). The problem varies relatively little by location or socioeconomic characteristics. Urban obesity rates are somewhat higher than rural (16.4 percent compared to 12.1 percent), and those among the non-poor are higher than those of the poor (16.1 percent compared to 13.3 percent). However, the incidence of obesity is strikingly lower than the average among indigenous mothers (7.4 percent, half the average level of 14.6 percent).

Ecuadorian women are also, on average, short: 13.7 percent are below the height benchmark of 1.45 meters normally used to define adult stunting (Table 13). Almost half of these short women are also overweight: 5.9 percent of women aged 15-45 are both stunted (below 1.45 meters) and overweight, and a further 2.1 percent are obese and overweight. This is consistent with international evidence that poor nutrition in early life can predispose individuals to obesity, heart disease, and diabetes in adulthood. It follows that addressing stunting in young children can help prevent other forms of malnutrition and noncommunicable disease in later life (see Box 3).

Maternal Nutrition and Children's Stunting. Small mothers are more likely to have children who are small. As can be seen in Figure 17, this relationship holds true in Ecuador, for both indigenous and nonindigenous women. The transmission is likely to come through the physical constraint on intrauterine growth during pregnancy—but maternal health problems, linked to the problems of overweight among smaller women, are also likely to be part of the story.

The coexistence of maternal overweight and children's stunting is sometimes known as the "double burden of disease." Some 24 percent of Ecuadorian households with a stunted child have overweight mothers, and 19 percent have obese mothers (Table 14).

This coexistence of cases of child undernutrition and adult overweight within the same family has also been observed in other countries. Studies of this phenomenon suggest

---

15. Type 2: non-insulin-dependent.

16. For adults, the BMI is the preferred indicator of nutritional status, because it is considered a better indicator of adequate nutritional status for adults than height-for-age, which reflects the composite interaction of feeding practices and morbidity history. See Appendix B for a fuller discussion of BMI.

Table 12. Maternal Weight Sufficiency in Ecuador

| | % of mothers who are | | | |
	Under-weight	Normal weight	Over-weight	Obese
Indigenous	0.4	52.4	39.9	7.4
Mestizo	2.0	42.0	40.9	15.1
White	2.3	42.5	37.3	17.9
Black	2.9	45.6	36.3	15.3
Urban	2.1	41.1	40.4	16.4
Rural	1.6	45.9	40.4	12.1
Sierra	1.1	44.7	41.8	12.4
Costa	2.5	41.2	39.8	16.5
Amazonia	2.4	47.6	35.0	15.0
Insular	0.0	38.4	44.2	17.4
Q1	2.7	46.1	38.2	13.0
Q2	2.6	45.3	38.3	13.8
Q3	1.2	42.3	41.8	14.7
Q4	1.0	39.0	41.8	18.2
Q5	0.5	36.8	47.1	15.6
Poor	2.6	45.7	38.3	13.3
Non-poor	1.0	40.0	43.0	16.1
Total	**1.9**	**43.1**	**40.4**	**14.6**

Note: Underweight BMI < 18.5. Normal:18.5 > BMI < 25. Overweight: 25 < BMI > 30. Obese BMI >= 30.0. Excludes pregnant women.
Source: World Bank calculation using ENDEMAIN 2004.

that it reflects a complex physiological interaction between childhood stunting and the production of adult obesity—so that small girls are likely to become obese women—coupled with the fact that small women are also more likely to have stunted children (due to intrauterine growth constraints and a higher prevalence of maternal morbidity). Box 3 summarizes the literature on this point.

Table 13. Stunting and Overweight in Adult Women

	Under-weight	Normal weight	Over-weight	Obese	Total
Height	Percentage of women aged 15–45				
>1.45 m	1.7	37.6	34.5	12.5	86.3
<1.45 m	0.2	5.5	5.9	2.1	13.7
Total	**1.9**	**43.1**	**40.4**	**14.6**	**100.0**

Note: 1.45 meters is the cutoff point below which an adult woman is considered stunted.
Source: World Bank, using ENDEMAIN 2004.

Box 3: Why Do Many Stunted Children Have Overweight Mothers?

The changing face of malnutrition, resulting from changes in diet, activity patterns, health, and nutrition is known as the "nutrition transition." As incomes rise and populations become more urban, shifts occur from energy-intensive work and traditional high-fiber, starch-based diets to more sedentary work and diets higher in fat and energy. This results in increased rates of obesity, and with it, nutrition-related noncommunicable diseases (HNP 2002). In general in developing countries, urban areas suffer more acutely from the nutrition transition than their rural counterparts, although rural problems of overweight and obesity are increasing.

According to WHO, obesity is increasing worldwide at an alarming rate, for both children and adults. Child obesity is an important predictor of adult obesity—about one-third of obese preschool children and one-half of school-age children grow up to be obese adults. Obesity leads to the development of diabetes, hypertension, stroke, cardiovascular disease, and some forms of cancer (Martorell 2001).

As in developed countries, in many developing countries, obesity is no longer a distinguishing feature of high socioeconomic status, but instead is itself becoming a marker of poverty. The Middle East, the Western Pacific, and Latin America show far higher levels of obesity than other developing regions (Popkin 2000). And obesity in developing countries is growing quickly. This is due, in part, to cheap edible oils and sugar consumption, which have increased fat and energy intake dramatically (HNP 2002). In Latin America and the Caribbean, oil per capita availability more than tripled during 1961–2000, while food from animal sources increased by about 50 percent (SNC 2004; Popkin 2004; Doak 2002).

In Latin America, a striking dimension of the nutrition transition is the association between obesity and stunting. Children who become stunted, due to nutritional failure during pregnancy or early life, face a higher risk of developing obesity later in life, because they become "programmed" to conserve fat and thus oxidize fat poorly, leading in turn to greater vulnerability to chronic, noncommunicable diseases in adulthood (Forsdal 1977; Barker 1992, 1994; HNP 2002; Branca 2002). This phenomenon, known as the Barker Hypothesis, helps to explain the coexistence of a stunted child with an overweight mother, known as SCOWT. A recent IFPRI study found a SCOWT prevalence of 11 percent in Bolivia, 13 percent in Guatemala, and 10 percent in Nicaragua. Intensified efforts are needed to reduce maternal malnutrition, improve pregnancy outcomes, and reduce early childhood stunting (thereby reducing that portion of adult obesity stemming from early deprivation). At the same time, increased attention to food quality (and particularly to fat and sugar intake) is needed, to address the portion of adult obesity which is diet related (Garrett and Ruel 2003).

Figure 17. The Relationship between Mothers' Height and Child's Height in Ecuador

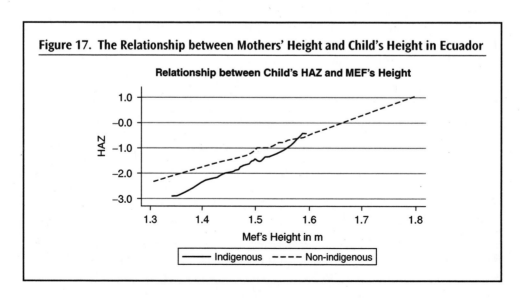

Table 14. Prevalence of Child stunting in Households with Overweight Mothers (% of households)

	Overweight Mother	Obese Mother
Indigenous	54.9	57.6
Mestizo	22.1	17.8
White	20.2	13.3
Black	14.7	15.6
Urban	18.2	16.5
Rural	33.0	24.2
Sierra	31.8	31.4
Costa	18.0	10.9
Amazonia	19.5	23.5
Insular	9.4	14.3
Poor	31.7	24.5
Non-poor	16.7	14.4
Total	24.2	19.2

Note: Overweight people are defined as having BMI levels between 25.0 and 29. Obesity is levels of BMI $> = 30.0$. Nonpregnant women only.

Source: World Bank, using ENDEMAIN 2004.

Behavior that Affects Nutritional Outcomes in Ecuador: Qualitative and Quantitative Evidence

Statistical Evidence on the Behavioral Correlates of Stunting

It is difficult to estimate the impact of behavioral variables such as breast-feeding and attendance at health posts on stunting outcomes in a cross-sectional analysis, due to the problem of "endogeneity" (or inverse causality). For instance, a mother might be more inclined to breast-feed her child because she has become aware that it is not growing properly, and she may be more likely to take a child to the health post if she realizes it is not growing properly. Similarly, the feedback loop which makes malnourished children more vulnerable to sickness makes it hard to precisely specify causality in that relationship.

In all of these cases, a simple cross-sectional analysis which correlates the child's nutritional status with the mother's behavior (without the benefit of a rigorously defined comparison or control group) is unlikely to capture the real impact of positive behaviors on nutritional outcomes. For this reason, such variables were excluded from the econometric analysis presented in the previous section.

Nevertheless, it has been well-established, in rigorous international studies, that exclusive breast-feeding in the first six months of life, regular attendance at child growth clinics and nutrition advice sessions, the institutionalization of births, and the avoidance (and proper management of) diarrheas, will all contribute to improved growth outcomes. The ENDEMAIN data set confirms that such behaviors tend to be associated with better nutritional outcomes in Ecuador, as detailed in the following sections.

Box 4: Breast-feeding: The Lessons of International Experience

The benefits of exclusive breast-feeding in the first six months of life have been confirmed in many studies. A 1984 "meta-analysis" (reference) concluded that exclusive breast-feeding from birth to 4-6 months significantly protects children against death by infectious disease. Breast-feeding results in higher immunological and emotional benefits to the infant, and in higher rates of intelligence, visual acuity, and lower blood pressure among 13–16 year olds. Benefits to mothers who breast-feed include extended postpartum infertility (leading to greater birth spacing), and a lower likelihood of contracting breast and ovarian cancer.

In spite of this evidence, the prevalence of breastfeeding has declined over the past several decades in developing countries, due to poor understanding of doctors, coupled with the commercial promotion of breast milk substitutes, and the fear of mother-to-child HIV transmission. This trend places a premium on devising effective promotional strategies. Some that have worked well are the following:

- *Philippines:* Hospital-based breast-feeding promotion—prohibiting the use of bottles, allowing "rooming-in" of infants with their mothers, using breast milk for sick and premature infants, offering breast-feeding counseling and support for mothers, and providing training for health care workers—led to increased breast-feeding rates and a sharp reduction in infant mortality.

- *Canada:* The distribution of breast-feeding promotion kits in hospitals, including information for physicians, resulted in an increase in breast-feeding prevalence from 25 percent during 1965—71 to 69 percent by 1982.

- *Papua New Guinea:* Breast-feeding promotion included a school-based breast-feeding promotion campaign and government regulations on the sales of bottles, pacifiers, and artificial nipples, and a ban on commercial advertising of breast milk substitutes. Only with a doctor's prescription can a mother purchase a feeding bottle. Breast-feeding rates increased as a result.

- *Brazil:* Brazil achieved an increase in exclusive breast-feeding from 3.8 percent in 1986 to 35.6 percent in 1996. PNIAM, Brazil's national breast-feeding program, has provided national coordination and support for state- and community-level initiatives and supported social mobilization including TV commercials during soap operas, and messages on lottery tickets and water, electricity, and telephone bills, and personal bank account statements. With support from the Catholic Church, the literacy movement, mothers' groups and professional associations, a breast-feeding promotion office was established in each state. Human-milk-bank committees were established, which collected, processed, and stored breast milk for distribution to needy infants. Labor legislation was amended to include benefits in support of breast-feeding: women were given the right to a 4-month maternity leave to facilitate exclusive breast-feeding and men were given the right to 5 days of paternity leave to support the mother in the critical period of starting breast-feeding. In 2002, the country launched a new campaign to promote breast-feeding in basic health units and complement Baby Friendly Hospitals.

Internationally, there is a growing recognition of the nutritional benefits of breast-feeding—as reflected, for example, in the recent Lancet Child Survival Series, which showed breast-feeding to be the most effective preventive intervention in preventing child mortality. This has led to the adoption of the International Code of Marketing of Breast-milk Substitutes and of the Baby Friendly Hospital Initiative (BFHI), two major policy actions in support of breast-feeding. In line with this consensus, in 2007, **Ecuador** plans to inaugurate its first breast milk bank and center for promoting breast-feeding in the Quito maternity and children's hospital.

Feeding Knowledge and Practices. The positive association between exclusive breast-feeding up to 6 months of age and infant growth is well documented in the literature (Castillo 1996; Victora and others 1984). Breast milk has adequate nutrition properties and also contains antibodies that protect children against illness. Breast-feeding also lengthens postpartum infertility, widening birth intervals (Box 4).

Breast-feeding is a common practice in Ecuador. Data from ENDEMAIN show that 95.7 percent of babies aged under 6 months are breast-fed; of these, 39.6 percent are exclusively breast-fed. The prevalence of exclusive breast-feeding is higher than average in the Sierra region, among indigenous women and among women from poor households.

Breast-feeding counseling is associated with lower stunting rates (about 10 percentage points lower, on average). The most important reductions in malnutrition associated with counseling are observed in rural areas, in the Sierra and among the poorest households (Table 15).

Prenatal Care, Birth Attendance, and Birth Weight. Stunting rates are much lower for children whose mother received prenatal care—and the greater the number of visits, the lower the prevalence of malnutrition. As would be expected, malnutrition rates are also much lower for children whose mother attended prenatal control in private clinics or social security clinics (Table 16).

Malnutrition rates are much higher for children who were born at home: the stunting rate for home-born children is 37.8 percent, compared with 18.6 percent for those born in institutional settings (Table 17). This holds even when controlling for location, ethnicity,

Table 15. Proportion of Stunted Children by Whether Their Mother Had Breast-feeding Counseling

	Received Counseling	Not Received Counseling	Total
Indigenous	32.6	45.7	42.7
Mestizo	14.6	21.4	18.5
White	14.7	21.8	18.8
Black	6.9	16.0	11.9
Urban	12.3	17.7	15.2
Rural	20.8	30.4	27.3
Sierra	21.8	32.7	28.6
Costa	10.2	15.5	13.1
Amazonia	16.8	22.8	20.7
Insular	2.6	16.3	9.7
Poor	18.0	28.1	24.7
Non-poor	12.7	17.3	15.0
Total	15.2	24.0	20.4

Note: Numbers are estimated for the last child alive in the HH who was born after January 1999.
Source: World Bank calculation using ENDEMAIN 2004.

Table 16. Proportion of Stunted Children by Number and Type of Prenatal Controls

	Number of Controls			Type of Controls			
	No Control	1 to 5 Controls	>5 Controls	Public	Private	Social Sec.	Total
Indigenous	54.3	43.5	39.6	44.8	28.5	29.5	46.5
Mestizo	31.6	26.4	16.9	23	14	14	21
White	31	26.6	15.1	21.1	9	16.7	18.8
Black	21.2	24.8	8.7	14.4	12	0	14.5
Urban	27.8	22.1	14.2	20.2	10.3	11	16.9
Rural	40.7	33.9	22.9	29	24.3	19.2	30.5
Sierra	43.9	39.3	24	33.5	22	16.5	31.9
Costa	28.1	17.6	12.7	17.2	9.1	7.9	15.6
Amazonia	30.9	32.3	12.4	22.3	17.5	22.2	22.8
Insular	0	50	8	10	5.5	0	8.4
Poor	39.3	29.7	21.3	26.4	19.4	21.4	27.6
Non-poor	26.1	26.7	13.4	20.4	11	11.5	16.4
Total	36.6	29	17.1	24.5	14	14.1	23.1

Source: World Bank calculation using ENDEMAIN 2004.

and poverty levels: the ratio is almost 2 to 1 in most cases. This suggests that high importance should be attached to increasing the institutional coverage of births, where mothers
are more likely to receive guidance on care and feeding practices and children are more
likely to receive immediate care and immunizations.

Table 17. Proportion of Stunted Children by Place of Birth Attendance

	Birth at Home	Birth other Place	Total
Indigenous	50.2	39.6	46.6
Mestizo	34.1	18.1	21.1
White	35	15.7	18.6
Black	17.9	13.4	14.2
Urban	27.9	15.8	16.9
Rural	40.6	23.9	30.6
Sierra	46.9	25.3	31.9
Costa	25.2	13.9	15.6
Amazonia	26.8	20.8	22.7
Insular	—	7.5	8.4
Poor	37.9	22.4	27.6
Non-poor	37.2	14.7	16.5
Total	37.8	18.6	23.1

Source: World Bank calculation using ENDEMAIN 2004-CEPAR—Ecuador.

Table 18. Proportion of Stunted Children by Whether they were Weighed at Birth, and by Sufficiency of Weight at Birth

	Weighed	Not weighed	Low weight at birth	High weight at birth	Total
Indigenous	46.4	50.1	59.5	39.1	48.1
Mestizo	19.4	33.4	30.6	16.8	21.5
White	17.8	27.3	25.4	17.2	19
Black	12.7	24.4	28.6	9.2	14.8
Urban	16.4	27	27.5	13.8	17.2
Rural	27.7	40	39.6	24.2	31.5
Sierra	28.2	47.4	36.7	25.1	32.5
Costa	15	22.5	27.1	12.3	16
Amazonia	20.1	32.7	42.9	16.4	23.4
Insular	7.9	0	0	7.2	7.6
Poor	25.1	37.2	38.4	21.3	28.3
Non-poor	15.6	34.7	24	13.8	16.8
Total	**20.7**	**36.8**	**32.4**	**17.6**	**23.6**

Note: Low weight at birth refers is less than 5.5 lbs. If there is no record of the weight at birth, the survey asks the mothers if the child weighted less than 5.5 lbs.
Source: World Bank calculation using ENDEMAIN 2004.

As noted above, the ENDEMAIN study includes data on whether the child was weighed at birth, and on birth-weight sufficiency.[17] Having been weighed at birth is an indicator of the mother's take-up of recommended protocols. Birth weight itself is an indicator of nutrient intake during the fetal period; previous studies have shown an association between low birth weight and higher risks of death (Habicth and others 1973), and between low birth weight and the likelihood of becoming stunted.

The ENDEMAIN data indicate that the probability of being stunted is much higher for children who were not weighed at birth, compared with those who were weighed (37 percent compared to 21 percent); and among those who were weighed, it is higher for those born with low birth weight (defined as lower than 2,500 grams), compared with those born with sufficient birth weight (32.4 percent compared to 17.6 percent). These differences hold independently of ethnicity, location, or income levels (Table 18).

The relationship between the height-for-age z-score and birth weight for children who had a written record available, is plotted in Figure 18. It can be seen that stunted children report lower birth weights, compared with those who are not stunted (the distribution of the density function is shifted to the left). The dotted vertical line indicates the cutoff point for the conventional definition of low birth weight (5.5 lbs).

---

17. These data should be interpreted with care, because they are based on mothers' recollection. When the mother could not remember the actual weight, she was asked to state whether it was low birth weight, or not.

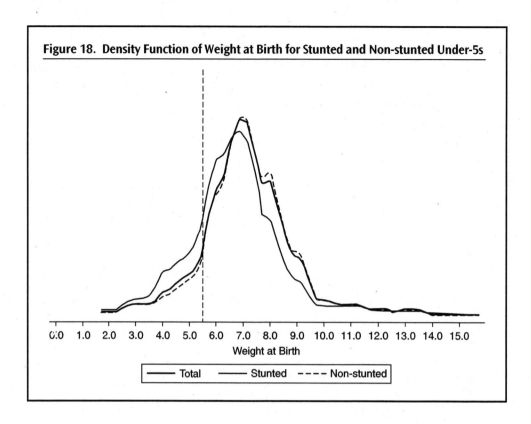

Figure 18. Density Function of Weight at Birth for Stunted and Non-stunted Under-5s

Postnatal Controls, Infections, and Health Practices. Infectious diseases such as diarrhea and acute respiratory infections negatively affect a child's nutritional status by diminishing appetite and reducing the absorption, utilization, and requirements of nutrients. Diarrhea is one of the most important diseases to affect nutritional status, and the risk of diarrhea is at its highest during the termination of breast-feeding (Pebely, Hurtado, and Goldman 1999; *Journal of Biosocial Sciences*). Nutritional status is affected through loss of appetite, vomiting, energy loss during fever, and other factors (Rohde 1986; Victora and others 1986).

For these reasons, attendance at postnatal clinics and the application of full immunization protocols are important factors affecting nutritional outcomes. The data from ENDE-MAIN indicate that these relationships are valid in Ecuador, as in other countries. Table 19 shows that children who have attended postnatal controls are less likely to be stunted than those who have not done so, and that children who use health ministry facilities (normally those from more vulnerable backgrounds) have higher stunting rates than others.

Similarly, children in Ecuador who have had diarrhea and acute respiratory infections are much more likely to be stunted than those who have not. However, this is not a unidirectional relationship. It is complicated by the feedback mechanism between illness and stunting. A child whose nutritional status has been weakened by past episodes of illness becomes in turn more prone to illness in the future. Table 20 shows that, nationwide, stunting stood at 28.5 percent among children who suffered from diarrhea in the last two weeks, compared with 20.8 percent for those who did not. This holds good across socioeconomic categories. The relationship of stunting to acute respiratory infections is much less clear, however. The reported difference of 1.5 percentage points is within the margin of error for the estimation.

Table 19. Proportion of Stunted Children by Attendance at Postnatal Clinics and Type of Facility Used

| | Attendance at clinics | | Type of facility | | | |
	Yes	No	Public	Private	Social sec.	Total
Indigenous	53.3	39.6	53.1	69.1	27.4	53.3
Mestizo	21	16.7	24.8	9.6	6.4	21.1
White	17.7	12.1	19.8	8.6	18.7	17.8
Black	17.1	7.9	20.5	0	0	17.6
Urban	17.7	14	21.4	10.1	8.4	17.9
Rural	31.6	22.9	33.7	14.2	8.9	31.7
Poor	29	21.2	31.1	11.9 ·	16.7	29.2
Non-poor	17.5	10.1	21.9	10.6	4.9	17.6
Total	**24**	**17.7**	**27.8**	**10.9**	**8.6**	**24.2**

Note: Estimated for one selected child in each HH.
Source: World Bank calculation using ENDEMAIN 2004.

Immunization. The presence of an immunization register within the household seems to make little difference to stunting levels. This is probably due to the fact that many mothers of adequately immunized children did not have their records at hand. However, among those with records at hand, there is a clear positive influence of immunization sufficiency

Table 20. Proportion of Children Who Are Stunted, by their Exposure to Diarrhea and Acute Respiratory Infections

	Diarrhea	No Diarrhea	ARI	No ARI	Total
Indigenous	61.2	46.9	58.5	46.3	50.7
Mestizo	23.9	18.8	19.1	20.4	19.9
White	26	14	9.7	22.7	16.2
Black	22.7	12	16.9	11.9	14.8
Urban	19.5	15.9	17.5	15.9	16.6
Rural	38.5	27	27.4	31.1	29.6
Sierra	41.1	29.6	31.6	32.6	32.2
Costa	17.5	13.1	14.9	13.1	14.1
Amazonia	21.1	23.7	31	21.1	23.1
Insular	12.5	9.2	0	11	9.5
Poor	32.5	25	25.8	27.4	26.7
Non-poor	21.2	15	15	17	16.2
Total	**28.5**	**20.8**	**21.6**	**23.1**	**22.5**

Note: Numbers are estimated for a selected child alive in the HH.
Source: World Bank calculation using ENDEMAIN 2004-CEPAR—Ecuador.

Table 21. Proportion of Children Who Are Stunted, by Immunization Status

	Has carnet	Has no carnet	Complete immunization	Incomplete immunization
Urban	19.9	18.1	17.6	23.3
Rural	32.7	38.4	32.5	38.9
Poor	30.2	33.1	28.9	35.1
Non-poor	19	18.8	17.7	22.6
Total	**25.5**	**27.3**	**23.8**	**31.1**

Source: World Bank calculation using ENDEMAIN 2004.

on nutritional status: stunting rates are 23.8 percent compared with 31.1 percent for those with the protocol incomplete (Table 21).

Food Consumption. The highest rates of chronic malnutrition in Ecuador are concentrated in the rural Sierra, among the poorest and indigenous population. The international literature on the linkages from altitude to stunting (see Box 1 presented previously) suggests that dietary insufficiency-resulting in micronutrient deficiencies-is likely to be an important part of the cause. To investigate this hypothesis, this section analyzes food consumption data from ENDEMAIN, presenting data on consumption patterns of the main food elements, like meat, dairy, eggs, cereals, tubers, vegetables, and fruit. Although the data have limitations,[18] it is possible to estimate the monetary value of per capita consumption of the main food groups (including food grown at home or on the interviewee's farm) by region, altitude levels, and consumption quintiles.

The data from ENDEMAIN suggest that the problem of stunting in Ecuador is not primarily related to the lack of capacity to buy food. Once the data are broken down by income quintile or other socioeconomic categories, it can be seen that food consumption in the homes of stunted children is very similar to that for non-stunted children's homes. This is observed both in the subset of the survey sample where a detailed ("large") expenditure questionnaire was applied, and in those which responded to a "short" expenditure questionnaire. Nor does the proportion of food expenditure in total expenditure vary markedly between the homes of stunted and non-stunted children (Table 22).

The relationship between food expenditure and total expenditure behaves as is normally expected: in the bottom end of the income distribution there is a high elasticity of food spending to total spending, but this declines as food sufficiency levels are reached and food expenditure then becomes income inelastic. This is illustrated in Figure 19 (based on the short consumption questionnaire, for which there are more observations).

---

18. The main limitation is that the value of food products has important regional variations that cannot be unraveled in the data due to the lack of quantity registers. As a result, the difference in the amount of consumption between the poor and non-poor is likely to be understated, because the price of food is generally higher in more remote areas. However, this caveat does not invalidate the conclusions stated in the text.

Table 22. Average Per Capita Annual Household Food Consumption Expenditure (in $) by Child's Nutritional Status

	Long questionnaire		Short questionnaire		Food cons./Total exp.	
	Stunted	Non-stunted	Stunted	Non-stunted	Stunted	Non-stunted
Indigenous	488.7	455.4	402.2	380.6	51.9	48.7
Mestizo	520.5	636.6	479.5	521.7	48.7	45.1
White	537.2	845.9	464.9	592.4	44.3	46.8
Black	586.4	535.9	469.5	483.7	53.7	47.7
Urban	574.3	673.4	532.9	584.0	44.2	42.2
Rural	483.2	569.3	414.3	414.2	52.6	50.6
Sierra	513.3	628.5	472.0	508.5	46.8	41.4
Costa	536.8	643.3	447.5	529.9	53.7	49.2
Amazonia	375.1	544.1	465.7	418.9	48.4	40.2
Insular	404.7	740.8	308.8	571.1	22.0	33.5
Q1	326.10	327.50	275.70	285.20	54.40	52.40
Q2	541.60	534.70	463.10	451.80	50.30	49.40
Q3	757.00	714.50	559.40	588.80	44.20	44.60
Q4	770.10	940.20	745.70	771.30	37.90	39.10
Q5	1338.40	1037.20	1274.70	949.10	33.50	25.60
Poor	400.00	424.80	347.90	358.00	52.80	51.00
Non-poor	818.30	871.50	739.90	718.50	40.40	38.70
0–1,499 m.	534.50	639.90	441.30	511.20	53.30	48.40
1,500–2,499 m.	484.30	675.60	458.00	506.00	51.20	46.10
> 2,499 m.	508.10	615.10	493.20	540.20	44.50	38.90
Total	516.8	631.9	463.4	514.6	49.2	45.6

Source: World Bank calculation using ENDEMAIN 2004.

Detailed analysis of food expenditure by type also indicates that the *composition* of food expenditure is very similar between the homes of stunted and non-stunted children (Table 23). However, it is also noteworthy that the share of meat in total consumption is relatively low for households with stunted children at high altitudes (about 12 percent, compared with the general average of 18 percent). These data therefore support the hypothesis that a relative insufficiency of animal protein in the diet may be a cause of stunting in some regions of Ecuador.

Cultural Determinants of Diet and Health Practices in Ecuador

Given the decisive role of behavioral factors in determining nutritional outcomes, it is important to understand patterns of behavior and their cultural determinants. Ecuador has a rich and complex cultural tapestry, including a significant indigenous (Amerindian)

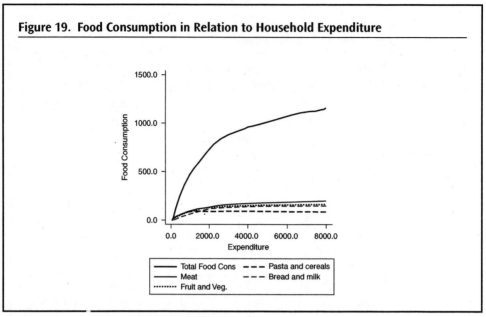

Figure 19. Food Consumption in Relation to Household Expenditure

Source: World Bank calculation using ENDEMAIN 2004.

population concentrated in the highlands and in the Amazon lowlands; and an important Afro-Ecuadorian population, descended from slaves, living mainly in coastal areas. There is also a large (mainly rural) population of culturally and racially *mestizo people*, who combine European and indigenous traits.

In this setting, traditional beliefs and behaviors might lead to feeding and health-care practices which are inimical to optimal growth outcomes and which may help to account for the poor nutritional status observed in rural and indigenous populations. Taking account of such beliefs and behaviors is an important dimension of the design of nutritional strategy. Service protocols may need to be adapted to maximize their acceptability to such groups, and educational programs will need to be designed to overcome resistance to key messages.

This subsection discusses cultural traits relevant to nutritional outcomes in Ecuador, based on a review of the relevant ethnographic, sociological, and anthropological literature, undertaken especially for this study, and makes recommendations for appropriate policy responses. Most of the literature reviewed here focuses on the indigenous inhabitants of the highlands and the Amazonian lowlands. Less has been written about the Afro-Ecuadorian population, which is primarily concentrated in the northwestern province of Esmeraldas and the valley of Chota in the northern highland province of Imbabura.

Overview of Relevant Beliefs and Practices. Knowledge, attitudes, and practices related to nutrition and health among Ecuador's indigenous and Afro-Ecuadorian communities involve two interrelated concepts: the differentiation between illnesses considered to be of natural or supernatural origin; and a set of dichotomies that explain and link the underlying nature of all things, including the origin of illnesses and their treatment. The most

Table 23. Share in Total Food Consumption of Different Types of Food (%)

	Bread and milk/Food cons			Meat/Food cons			Pasta and cereals/Food cons			Veg. and fruits/Food cons		
	Stunted	Non-stunted	Total	Stunted	Non-stunted	Total	Stunted	Non-stunted	Total	Stunted	Non-stunted	Total
Indigenous	12.3	12.3	12.3	12.8	15.6	14.3	16.1	12.4	14.2	22.9	21.1	21.9
Mestizo	14.2	14.5	14.4	17.2	19.1	18.7	12.7	12.0	12.2	18.6	18.6	18.6
White	17.1	14.7	15.2	13.8	19.8	18.7	10.5	11.2	11.0	21.0	21.3	21.2
Black	15.5	15.6	15.6	16.6	20.3	19.8	19.5	14.5	15.2	13.9	15.5	15.3
Urban	16.3	15.6	15.7	18.2	19.7	19.4	11.1	10.7	10.8	18.7	18.5	18.6
Rural	12.4	12.8	12.7	14.8	17.9	16.9	15.1	14.2	14.5	19.9	19.1	19.3
Sierra	16.6	18.5	17.9	12.6	15.3	14.4	13.3	11.8	12.3	20.3	19.1	19.5
Costa	10.3	11.6	11.4	23.0	22.1	22.2	13.9	12.6	12.8	18.5	18.6	18.6
Amazonia	9.1	15.0	13.7	12.8	13.4	13.3	13.3	10.8	11.3	16.2	18.3	17.8
Insular	16.1	15.9	15.9	19.8	19.6	19.6	1.9	5.6	5.3	17.6	18.8	18.7
Poor	12.2	12.7	12.6	16.0	19.0	18.2	15.3	14.3	14.5	19.9	18.8	19.1
Non-poor	18.2	16.6	16.9	16.5	18.9	18.5	9.2	9.4	9.4	18.3	18.7	18.6
0–1,499 m.	10.8	12.0	11.8	20.6	20.8	20.8	14.0	12.6	12.8	17.9	18.8	18.7
1,500–2,499 m.	13.6	17.0	15.8	11.5	14.2	13.3	15.5	12.6	13.6	18.1	18.0	18.0
> 2,499 m.	17.4	20.3	19.3	12.7	15.4	14.4	12.6	10.9	11.5	21.4	19.3	20.0
Total	**14.0**	**14.4**	**14.3**	**16.2**	**18.9**	**18.3**	**13.5**	**12.1**	**12.5**	**19.4**	**18.8**	**18.9**

Source: World Bank calculation using ENDEMAIN 2004.

important dichotomy refers to the concept of hot and cold, which is unrelated to temperature but is, rather, based on an understanding of the essential nature of virtually everything found in nature, including plants used for food, beverages, or remedies, and the human body itself. Other dichotomies include balance and lack of balance, strength and weakness, hard and soft, and masculine and feminine.

The concept of dichotomy is essential to the understanding of health and illness in general, and diet, in particular. Disequilibria in the hot-cold dichotomy are regarded in indigenous communities as the basis of illness and are believed to have a variety of origins (Balladelli and Colcha 1996; Hess 1994; Muñoz B. 1999). These beliefs also shape knowledge, attitudes, and practices of some rural and urban *mestizos* and whites (Argüello 1988; Uzendoski 2005); medicinal plants and herbs can be found in virtually any urban popular market and in elite shopping centers.

Indigenous and Afro-American communities have traditionally believed in the supernatural origin of some (but not all) maladies; among the most important are *mal aire, mal de ojo, espanto, and susto.* The origin attributed to them varies among different groups, but they have in common that they are found in nature, and may also involve either a spirit world or malevolent people or intentions. Similarly, treatments or cures practiced by traditional healers among—and even within—communities may differ, but in general, they involve herbal remedies.

Children are viewed as being particularly vulnerable to supernatural maladies because they are not as strong as adults and their personalities are viewed as incompletely formed. Women are sometimes regarded as having less strength (*fuerza*) than men. Some supernatural maladies are thought to befall evil people (*persona sinestra or lapiza* in the kichwa[19] language), or to be caused by aggressive behavior, egoism, or a false heart. In contrast, people with a good spirit or a good heart are not thought to be vulnerable to attacks by spirits. Finally, in this framework, it is possible to be bewitched through *brujería* (Argüello 1988; Balladelli and Colcha 1996; Hess 1994; Muñoz B. 1999; Uzendoski 2005).

Within this belief system, in general, the way to avoid illness is to lead a correct life, especially with respect to being sociable in the proper ways. Prosperity and health are achieved by maintaining an equilibrium (especially of temperature that is neither hot nor cold) and also a strong body and spirit. Bad luck is thought of as a malady attributable to disequilibria, which is remedied by trying to lead a good life marked by hard work; being peaceful, servile, and gentle with women, children, and parents; and participating in communal activities. Illness, in this context, is interpreted in terms of a spirit that is missing or out of balance.

Diet is also extremely important in this regard, because of the capacity to cause or correct disequilibria. This is because each food item is identified as hot or cold. The hot-cold equilibrium can be disturbed by eating too many rich foods, which are hot. Similarly, equilibrium can be reestablished by consuming the right food, beverage, or medicinal plant (Balladelli and Colcha 1996; Escobar K. 1990; Hess 1994; Muñoz B. 1999).

As noted above, though, not all illnesses are regarded as of supernatural origin. In some cases, ill health can be attributed to infection or other natural causes. The importance of

---

19. In this document, the term kichwa, now preferred in Ecuador, is used rather than the alternatives Quichua or Quechua to refer both to the indigenous group and their language.

Box 5: Supernatural Origin or Effects of Disease

"Pero hay muchachos pequeños que están ahí, como no sea de pegarles mal aire, no les pega. Pero cuando es de pegarle le pega, aun cuando el muchacho esté de este lado y el muerto esté del otro lado, le pega" (Escobar K. 1990:61). *"But there are small children around her; how can it be that the mal aire doesn't attack them; it doesn´t hit them. But when it does strike them, it does strike, even when the child is on this side and the dead person is on the other side, it strikes them."*

"No ve que el mal aire anda por la calle, vamos a decir, ese es como un espíritu, anda por la calle como un viento. Porque si usted va al cementerio, se pude decir que agarra mal aire ... bueno, porque estuvo donde los muertos. Pero fuera del cementerio, si es posible por medio del río le ataca, o si es posible lo ha tenido y contagiado y entonces se lo remueve. Puede ser como una cosa que se le pegue, como una peste que enteramente es como un viento (Escobar K. 1990:66). *"Don't you see that mal aire wanders in the street; let's say, it's like a spirit; it wanders the streets like a wind. Because if you go by a cemetery, you could say that the mal aire will attack you ... well, because you were where the dead are. But outside of the cemetery, it is possible to be attacked in the river, or it is possible that you've had it and been contaminated, and then you remove it. It can be like a thing that strikes, like a plague that is completely like a wind.*

Espanto hay de monte alto, espanto de muerto, espanto de agua y espanto de vivo. Son cuatro (Escobar K. 1990:71). *"There is* espanto *in the high mountain,* espanto *of the dead,* espanto *of water, and* espanto *of the living. There are four."*

---

this distinction is that it affects diet and health-seeking behavior. Muñoz B. (1999) and McKee (1988) document the perceived difference between illnesses that should be treated at home or by a traditional healer on one hand, and illnesses that should be treated by modern health practitioner, on the other.

This understanding of diet, health, and illness is reflected not only in health-related behaviors, but also in other spheres of everyday life, including farming systems. Gardens are an important element of indigenous agricultural systems, and while they offer multiple benefits, they are mostly devoted to the cultivation of medicinal plants. In essence, they are the medicine cabinet of the household, and they provide the family with the resources they need to treat illnesses of family members. Treatment is almost invariably provided by women. Plants with medicinal value can also be gathered in the wild. Finerman and Sackett (2003) show that Saraguro women (in the southern highland province of Loja) study their neighbor's home gardens in order to decipher the owners' economic and health status.

The Effect of Recent Socioeconomic Changes on Traditional Beliefs and Practices. The influence of traditional belief systems on the practices of indigenous and minority populations is shaped and constrained by Ecuador's economic, political, social, and ecological structures. Although there is an acceptance of the physical causes of some illnesses, and a concomitant belief in the effectiveness of modern therapies in treating them, the ability to access modern institutional health care services is conditioned by widespread poverty and exclusion. In the absence of effective access to modern services, people fall back on traditional alternatives. Similarly, access to an adequate diet (either through production or purchase) depends on agro-ecological conditions. In much of the highlands and Amazonian lowlands, access to land is limited in both quantitative terms (exacerbated by the intergenerational subdivision of historically small parcels) and qualitative terms because of poor agro-ecological characteristics (exacerbated by erosion and overexploitation of land that in many cases was marginal to begin with) (Sánchez-Parga 1984; Weismantel 1988).

The dramatic social, economic, and demographic changes of the past 20 years have altered the balance between modern and traditional belief systems. A generation ago, Ecuador was still essentially rural and agrarian, but today, two-thirds of the population live in urban areas. Urban-rural migration has resulted in dramatic changes in occupational structure, life styles, and the growth of the urban informal sector (Waters 1997). In this setting, traditional features of culture and forms of community organization have been weakened (Sánchez-Parga 1996). For example, traditional health practitioners are not being replaced and the younger generation increasingly holds to more "modern" health care ideas (Ruiz 1990). Moreover, the use of indigenous languages has been weakened by public education and mass media and by the increasingly widespread movement of people and ideas (Sánchez-Parga 1996). The accelerated trend of transnational migration that began in earnest after the financial and political crises of 2000 has taken a further toll on the cultural integrity of rural and indigenous communities (Herrera, Carrillo, and Torres 2005; Kyle 2000). The resulting decomposition of traditional structures has led to dysfunctional behavior patterns, such as alcoholism and domestic violence (Sanchez-Parga 1996) and of youth gangs, not only in urban settings, but even in small indigenous communities (Sozoranga 2006). Reactions to change are differentiated by gender and age; for example, older indigenous women have retained traditional cultural elements more than men, but there are signs of cultural erosion among the young (Guerrón 2000).

Notwithstanding these dramatic social and cultural changes, to indigenous people and Afro-Ecuadorians, the differences between themselves and the majority remain clear. Guerrón (2000) argues that Afro-Ecuadorians in the Chota valley of Imbabura province maintain their cultural identity with respect to other groups. More generally, the resurgence of the indigenous movement in Ecuador in the past 15 years is closely related to the continued vitality of ethnic and cultural identity (Albó 2004; Selverston-Scher 2001; Zamosc 2003). In this setting, ethnicity continues to shape nutrition and health-related knowledge, attitudes, and practices in Ecuador in many important ways. The following paragraphs explore, in more detail, culturally informed knowledge, attitudes, and practices of Ecuadorians related to nutrition and health, focusing on areas where service protocols might need culturally sensitive adjustments to promote the take-up of practices which would improve nutrition and health outcomes.

Traditional Diet. In highland indigenous communities, the traditional diet is poor and has little variation; grains (especially barley in the form of flour [*machica*] or roughly ground [*arroz de cebada*]), tubers (especially potatoes), and fava beans (*habas*) are the staples. Other grains (corn at lower altitudes and rice as an elite commodity) are consumed less often and fruit only occasionally (Weismantel 1988). Eggs and cheese are luxury goods in the highlands, and meat is usually consumed only during fiestas. The quality of the diet varies based on wealth and resource endowment (access to land, altitude, and soil type) and seasonal variations. In the rural highlands, food preparation time is limited because of scarcity of fuel (firewood); as a result, processed foodstuffs that require less time to cook—such as pasta—have tended to replace locally produced foods. Other processed foods include rolled oats (referred to as *quaker*), which is consumed as a beverage or used to thicken soups.

Box 6: Attitudes toward Family Size in Rural Areas of Pichincha Province

---

"Siempre es bueno tener guagüitos para el servicio, los hombrecitos van a trabajar y las mujerci-
tas ayudan en la casa, ayudan a cocinar, van a pastar, a traer leña." *"It is always good to have babies
to help out; the boys go to work and the girls help around the house, help in the cooking, to pasture
the animals, to bring firewood."*

"Hay que tener hijos, porque son una bendición de Dios para nosotros los pobres. Es bueno tener
los guagüitos, porque ayudan. Nosotros tenemos algunos animalitos y ellos van a pastar, les
cuidan." *"It is necessary to have children, because they are a blessing from God for us poor people. It
is good to have children, because they help out. We have some animals and they pasture them, take
care of them."*

"Con esto ya van a ser seis, con tal que Dios dé sano y salvo, sea hombre sea mujer, le recibiremos.
Nosotros tenemos granos en el campo, no es mucho, pero siempre hay para dar de comer." *"This
one will make six, so long as God makes it safe and sound; whether it be a boy or girl, we will receive
it. We have grain in the fields; it is not much, but there is always enough to eat."*

All quotes from: Estrella (1991:60).

In the Afro-Ecuadorian population, the diet is more varied and of better quality; the sta-
ple foodstuff is the plantain (consumed green, ripe, or dried and converted into flour), white
rice is consumed and there is more frequent consumption of animal-based protein: fish, wild
animals that are still hunted, or domestic animals, especially pork (Weigel and Castro 2001).

Maternal Diet in Pregnancy and After Childbirth. There is little evidence of harmful,
culturally determined dietary practices during pregnancy. According to Estrella's (1991)
study of rural women (mostly indigenous) in Pichincha province, pregnant women should
avoid getting wet or cold and should avoid foods thought of as cold or those considered
"heavy." They should eat foods that are good sources of protein: meat (especially mutton),
eggs, milk, and cheese, but in moderation. A healthy diet is seen to benefit the unborn child
and the mother. Other behavioral restrictions include avoiding hard work, especially at the
end of the pregnancy, abstaining from sexual relations, and adhering to several harmless
admonitions related to the understanding of the supernatural: pregnant women should
avoid coming into contact or even seeing malformed children (because those characteristics can be passed onto the unborn baby) and should avoid hills and rainbows that are the
source of spirits that can attack pregnant women.

Other sources report that in the highlands, indigenous families believe that the new
mother should avoid eating pork or any food that has been stored. They should consume
chicken or chicken soup and hot chocolate, but care should be taken in consuming salt or
sweets. Other restrictions include not showering or washing hair for five days, staying in
bed as much as possible, and keeping protected from the wind (Muñoz 1986). Bianchi
(1993) reports that pregnant Shuar women in the Amazonian lowlands observe no real
dietary restrictions, although the diet should not be too hot or salty.

However, there are some practices that contradict modern dietary norms. Torres (2006)
reports that pregnant indigenous women in Machachi (in the southern part of the province
of Pichincha) do not eat foods that are considered to be "infected," including peanuts and
cabbage. In some indigenous communities, it is believed that the belly of pregnant women

---

Box 7: The Role of Traditional Midwives

Opinions vary regarding the role and importance of traditional midwives, traditional birth atten-
dants (TBAs; *parteras or comadronas*), and it is noteworthy that much of the relevant literature is
quite old.

Naranjo (1984) affirms that every community in the highlands of Imbabura province has at least
one TBA and that even when institutional care is available, indigenous families prefer to follow
traditional practices, especially with respect to giving birth at home. According to Muñoz (1986),
in Cañar province midwives are experienced and capable. Among lowland kichwas, the midwife
is also viewed as indispensable. But according to Ordóñez (2005), home births explain the continued high maternal mortality rate in Chimborazo. A recent article on childbirth among the lowland kichwas of Orellana province suggests that the role of *parteras* continues to be important,
due to lack of transport (many people in the region travel mostly by motorized canoes) and poor
access to health centers and subcenters (*El Comercio* 2006b).

In the Afro-Ecuadorian communities in Esmeraldas province, TBAs have also been common. They
are usually female, but Escobar (1990) provides an ethnography of an elderly male traditional
healer who reports assisting many births. Afro-Ecuadorian inhabitants of the Chota valley in
Imbabura province north of Quito, also recur to TBAs. As in the indigenous communities, the TBA
cuts the umbilical cord and washes and wraps the baby. But Herrera (2000) notes a decline in mid-
wifery in Afro-Ecuadorian communities. In a case study conducted in Esmeraldas province,
74 percent of births were in institutions and 26 percent were at home, whereas 15 years earlier,
these proportions were reversed.

---

could explode, so it is recommended to drink alcohol instead of water (Muñoz 1986). After
birth, lowland kichwa parents engage in fasting and strict control of other behavior, referred
to as *sasina*. Fasting is related to concepts of the flow of energy between visible and invisible
realms. It is believed that abstention feeds and strengthens the baby and avoids doing it dam-
age or jeopardizing its proper development (Uzendoski 2005).

Attitudes on Institutional vs. Traditional Methods of Giving Birth. Giving birth at home,
with or without a traditional birth attendant, remains common in rural Ecuador. The coverage of prenatal consultation and institutional births among indigenous women is much
lower than that for the rest of the population. This, in turn, almost certainly results in higher
maternal and infant mortality. The associated lack of prenatal controls also probably contributes to a higher incidence of low-birth-weight babies and (later) stunted children. It is
therefore important to understand to what extent the distancing of indigenous women from
institutional birthing services is the product of downright cultural resistance to giving birth in
an institutional setting, to what extent it is the product of unnecessarily inflexible cultural
insensitivity in institutional services, and to what extent it simply reflects access problems.

There is abundant evidence that the cultural insensitivity of institutional services is a
factor causing indigenous women to reject the service. Among the lowland kichwa, it is
believed that physicians "cut up" women too much (likely to be a reference to the practice
of episiotomy during birth and the high prevalence of cesarian sections). According to Naula
(2006), indigenous women feel uncomfortable with the requirement to disrobe and wait
alone in a cold room. It is very important for indigenous people that the family be nearby
during childbirth. Similarly, in Cañar Province, women did not want to disrobe in front of

a male doctor (Muñoz 1986). There is a strong perception that indigenous women are not respected and are mistreated by staff in health facilities. Language is also a barrier: very few doctors speak kichwa or any other indigenous language, and this gap extends to formal health care services. While many indigenous people speak Spanish, many others—especially women, the very young, and the very old—do not, or speak and understand it poorly.

Women are also concerned that institutional services will not allow them to give birth in the position traditionally adopted throughout the Andean region. Highland kichwa women give birth in a squatting position (*hincadas*), usually on the floor, and supported by a bench, chair, or a wall. Lowland kichwas also give birth in this position, and may have their hands tied to beams in the ceiling. Similarly, Shuar women give birth in a squatting position supported either by a horizontal pole set up for the purpose, or by the husband (Bianchi 1993).

The return of the placenta is also an important issue. Indigenous and Afro-Ecuadorians have a multiplicity of beliefs surrounding the disposal of the placenta. In Imbabura province, it is buried beneath the *tullpa* or hearth, symbolizing a place of warmth and fertility. In the Chota valley, also in Imbabura province, Afro-Ecuadorian families bury the placenta and the umbilical cord near the entrance to the home so that the newborn will not suffer from stomach aches (Naranjo 1984). Estrella (1991) found that families in Pichincha bury the placenta so that the mother and child will not fall ill. In Pindlin (Cañar province), the placenta is commonly thrown into a river, in the belief that this will prevent the mother feeling thirsty during lactation (Munoz 1986). So the non-return of the placenta is a clear disincentive to opting for an institutionalized birth.

Early Childhood Nutritional Practices. The ENDEMAIN survey documents indigenous women's strong attachment to breast-feeding. This is consistent with the sociological literature, which shows that exclusive breast-feeding is favored, in general, because

---

Box 8: Return of the Placenta

"La placenta algunas veces sale con el muchacho, ¿ no ve que ella es la compañía del muchacho? Ella está pegada con el muchacho, está prendida del ombligo de él . . . . Hay algunas que son m*s pequeñas, otras son gradísimas, media peligrosa es. Hay veces salen con el muchacho, sale con todo y otras sale el muchacho y se quedan ellas blindadas ahí, . . . esa es la peligrosa. Si sale el muchacho y no sale ella, haga de cuenta que todavía no ha parido la mujer" *"The placenta sometimes comes out with the baby. Don't you see that it is the companion of the baby? It is stuck to the baby, stuck to the navel . . . There are some [placentas] that are smaller, others are very big—that's quite dangerous. There are times that [the placenta] comes out with the baby, everything comes out; and other times that they are thicker, that is the dangerous one. If the baby comes out and [the placenta] doesn't, you have to realize that the mother hasn't given birth.* (Escobar K. 1990:84–5).

La placenta se entierra, no hay que dejar encima, tirada en el suelo, se espanta el niño y la madre le puede dar mal aire. Si le entierra, se podría dar a luz otra vez, sin dolor. *"The placenta is buried; it shouldn't be left above [the ground], thrown on the ground, it shocks the child and the mother can get 'bad air.' If it's buried, the next birth wont be painful."* (Estrella 1991:72)

La placenta enterramos, no vale botar en el suelo, porque se enfría y ese frío pasa a la madre y duele. *"We bury the placenta; it shouldn't be thrown away, because it gets cold and this cold passes to the mother, and it hurts."* (Estrella 1991:72)

Box 9: Dietary Restrictions After Childbirth

(According to a traditional birth attendant): "Según la gente y según el cuerpo, la dieta dura unas treinta días, o quince días o ocho días. Primero, tiene que estar acostada, después conforme va endurando el cuerpo, puede levantar poco a poco. Tiene que comer comidas calientes, no salir al frío, no meter la mano en el agua, no bañarse. . . . Después de treinta días ya se puede bañar, cocinando una hierbita de monte, que se llama pumamaqui. . . *According to the people and depending on the body, the diet lasts about thirty days, or fifteen days or eight days. First, one has to have bed rest; later, depending on how the body recovers, one can get up gradually. One has to eat hot foods, not go out in the cold, not put the hand in water, not bathe. . . . After thirty days, one can bathe, cooking a wild plant called pumamaqui.*" (Estrella 1990:74).

---

mothers' milk is free, and is known to be good for the child. There is no evidence that women in Ecuador regard colostrum (the first milk, immediately after childbirth, which is particularly rich in nutrients) is harmful (as is the case in some African countries).

There are many traditional beliefs on ways to improve lactation. Women in Gualeceo (Azuay province) believe that their breast milk can decrease if their backs get cold, if they are exposed to the wind or the sun, if they get wet, or if they eat "cold" foods. They also believe that they should not breast-feed when pregnant (Novotny 1986). In a highland indigenous community Pigott and Kolasa (1983) found that breastfeeding was nearly universal. Lactation is thought to be stimulated by foods such as milk, soup, meat, oats, and also vitamins. In the Afro-Ecuadorian population, mothers breast-feed for between six months and a year (Whitten 1992).

There is substantial variation in weaning practices. Leonard and others (2000) found that breast-feeding continues for less time on the coast (16 months) than in the highlands (25 months). But substantial variation is found in highland communities. Stansbury, Leonard, and DeWalt (2000) found that in Cotopaxi province, indigenous women continue breast-feeding for 24 months. In contrast, weaning in Chimborazo was found to start at 8 to 10 months, or when the mother becomes pregnant again (Muñoz 1986). Among Afro-Ecuadorians in coastal Esmeraldas, babies are generally breast-fed for a year. If a woman becomes pregnant, breast-feeding is suspended. Otherwise, weaning takes place gradually between 6 and 18 months (Whitten 1997).

In general, boys are breast-fed for longer than girls. According to McKee (1987), in the highland region, it is believed that sexual characteristics are transmitted through breast milk. According to one of McKee's informants, girls should not be breast-fed for more than one year, because it makes them "too fertile" while boys should not be breast-fed for more than two years, because that will make them *malcriados* (badly behaved). Another informant stated that if girls are breast-fed for too long, it makes them too strong and they will look for men and have many babies. Novotny (1988) and Estrella (1991) also report that boys are breast-fed for longer periods, because it is believed that strength is passed to the child through the milk, and it is important for boys to be strong.

Management of Early Childhood Illnesses. Indigenous communities have strongly held beliefs about how sick children should be treated, many of which run directly against the grain of modern best practice. According to McKee (1988) there are two types of illnesses that they believe should not be treated by a doctor: those of supernatural origin, which are potentially life threatening and should be cured through ritual healing; and those which are relatively minor and are treatable at home with plant remedies. Illnesses that should be treated by a doctor are those due to infection.

Home treatment of diarrhea usually includes withholding of food and liquids; the intake of liquids is believed to make the condition worse. If diarrhea is foamy or contains mucous, the illnesses is judged to be "cold." Treatment consists of warming the child. On the other hand, if the diarrhea is judged to be curdled (like sour milk), or green or yellow, the illness is considered to be supernatural. It might be the product of evil eye (*mal de ojo*), bad air (*mal aire*), or evil spirits (*espanto or susto*), and treatment will vary accordingly. In cases of mal aire treatment is by ritual cleaning, including rubbing the child with objects with an intense smell (Argüello 1988; McKee 1988). McKee found that in several highland provinces, mothers stop breast-feeding babies who are ill. Novotny (1988) also found that mothers in Gualaceo (Azuay province) believed that they should not breast-feed an ill child, and that children should not eat when sick, especially in cases of diarrhea.

The Decision to Use Formal Health Services. Notwithstanding the traditional beliefs documented in the preceding paragraphs, the sociological literature shows that indigenous Ecuadorians do not reject modern health care per se. Rather, they chose among options depending on the circumstances, taking account of culturally based perceptions about which illnesses should be treated in institutional settings and which are more appropriate for traditional care, and bearing in mind access conditions for modern services.

A 1982 study in highland kichwa communities and among Shuars and Achuars in the Amazonian lowlands provided data on 3,670 episodes of illness. Of these, half were treated at home, 27 percent with institutional health care, 10 percent by traditional healers, and 13 percent by pharmacists or drug sellers—a pattern which is similar to that observed in more recent health demand surveys. When consulted, many said they did not use institutional care because it was inaccessible or unaffordable; fully half of the respondents said that, given the choice, they would select it. Age, sex, primary education, and material assets did not influence the choice between institutional or traditional health care, but secondary education and access to modern health care did (Kroeger 1982a). Similarly, a study in the Amazon lowlands found that among the women of the Puyo Runa (kichwas in Pastaza province) the perceived barriers to institutional care were lack of time and money and the belief that services would not be available when needed. The cost of retrieving the body of someone who had died in a hospital was seen as a barrier to seeking institutional care (Whitten and Whitten 1985). The health events for which there is greatest reluctance to use institutionalized services are those associated with birth and death. Among Saraguro families, for example, childbirth is viewed as a private act, whereas they believe that in hospitals, it is converted into a public act (Finerman 1983, 1989).

This interplay between cultural preferences and economic barriers in determining the effective demand for institutional healthcare is not limited to Ecuador's indigenous population. A recent study of highland *mestizo* women in southern Azuay province identified the lack of financial resources as the principal barrier to access to formal health care, but also documented widespread acceptance of traditional practices and distrust of outsiders. These women rely extensively on traditional medicines, partly because they are free, but

Box 10: Community-based Child Development Programs-the AIN-C Program in Honduras

Experience in Latin America has shown that integral, community-based child development programs (*Atención Integral a la Ninez-Comunitaria*, AIN-C)—which couple nutritional counseling and growth monitoring with strong linkages to health service delivery—have the potential to improve nutrition outcomes in countries similar to Ecuador. AIN-C, which was first developed in Honduras, has inspired comparable programs in Bolivia, El Salvador, Ghana, Guatemala, Nicaragua, Uganda, and Zambia.

The AIN-C strategy is predicated on the idea that a large portion of child illness and malnutrition-related problems can be dealt with satisfactorily at the community level, and that this is more efficient than having the health post serve as the initial point of contact. It seeks to improve child health and nutrition by (a) improving child feeding and child care practices; (b) diagnosing, treating, and/or referring common illnesses; and (c) improving the use of existing health-related services. In Honduras, the program is managed by the Ministry of Health and implemented through NGOs in eight zones particularly prone to high stunting rates.

AIN-C builds on a long tradition of health-related volunteerism in Honduras. The focus is on children under the age of 2. Primary actors are the community volunteers, or *monitoras*, with an average of three *monitoras* responsible for 25 children (a much smaller ratio than is normally seen in such programs). The *monitoras* are better trained and far better equipped than community workers in most other programs. They use a modified Integrated Management of Childhood Illness (IMCI) protocol and are permitted to provide antibiotics to children. *Monitoras* visit newborns to enroll them in AIN within 48 hours of birth, and ensure a BCG vaccination is given. On average, *monitoras* devote about 15 hours per month, of which 4.5 hours is devoted to the monthly growth monitoring. AIN-C provides symbolic incentives (letters of thanks from senior officials, ID cards, parties honoring them).

The primary activities are monthly weighing sessions. At the end of each month *monitoras* aggregate individual growth data into bar graphs using five indicators (filling in vertical bars rather than calculating percentages): number of under 2s in the community, percent weighed, percent gaining adequate weight, percent with inadequate weight gain, and percent gaining inadequate weight for two or more months. AIN-C focuses on parents and on communities as the prime users of the data. The indicators serve as the basis for targeting home visits, focusing supervision, mobilizing community action, and for Health Ministry reporting.

Unlike Save the Children's positive deviance-based programs and related "hearth" programs, which concentrate on the rehabilitation of malnourished children, the focus of AIN-C is primarily on prevention. For this reason, less attention is paid to the nutritional "status" of the child and more to the *trajectory* of the child's growth curve. A healthy trajectory—even when the child is moderately malnourished—receives less attention from the *monitora* than a child of normal weight who fails to gain adequate weight from month to month. More attention also is given to assure understanding of growth curves by mothers or other caretakers.

The program's main strategy to improve nutrition and health is the promotion of behavioral change. Using the child's growth as the trigger for discussion, the *monitora* refers to counseling cards differentiated by child age, the adequacy or inadequacy of weight gain, health status, and breast-feeding status. She negotiates with the mother one change in her nurturing practices, to be carried out during the coming month. The next month, with updated growth information, the conversation continues, focusing initially on the negotiated change. A radio program also is broadcast to popularize key behaviors.

Synergies with the primary health system are strong. The nurse auxiliary from the closest Centro *de Salud Rural* (CESAR) attends growth monitoring sessions to update immunizations, distribute micronutrients and medications, arrange clinic appointments, and discuss family planning. AIN-C *monitoras* use IMCI protocols (originally developed for clinic use, but here adapted for community use). The *monitoras* are equipped with timers to diagnose pneumonia and antibiotics to treat it. The protocols provide for referral to the health post when a child is seriously ill or has persistent or acute growth failure. A "counter referral slip" is returned to the *monitora* from the health

---

**Box 10: Community-based Child Development Programs-the AIN-C Program
in Honduras (*Continued*)**

---

center, indicating the action taken and the community level follow-up necessary. *Monitoras* also
provide information on eligibility for and access to relevant services, including trash disposal, sanitation, the maintenance of community water sources, and emergency assistance.

However, the AIN-C experience also suggests that an effective community-based project requires
a strong health infrastructure for support and for dealing effectively with referrals. Between 1990
and 1996, the number of health centers in Honduras increased by 37 percent (World Bank 1997a).
Going forward, such programs should strengthen links with health centers—especially for height
monitoring of children over 12 months of age and referrals for morbidities—and there is also a
need for more rigorous impact evaluations.

---

also because it is widely believed that they work. Herbal teas (*aguitas*) are used to treat fever,
headaches, or urinary tract infections, and for illnesses regarded as originating in disequi-
librium in the hot-cold dichotomy. Other traditional methods include herbal tea baths and
limpiezas (ritual cleanings), in which an egg is passed over the body to diagnose maladies
of supernatural origin, such as *espanto* or *mal de ojo*. Only when traditional remedies do
not work are outsiders brought in. First, pharmacists are consulted for the purchase of
drugs. Doctors are consulted as a last option because of the perceived costs, which are
regarded as prohibitive (Schoenfeld and Jurabe 2005).

A critical additional factor limiting demand for modern services in rural areas and
marginal urban neighborhoods is the limited hours of clinic operation and low problem-
resolution capacity of the health post staff and facility, including a lack of basic medicines,
equipment, and materials (Platin 2003; Tigasi 2006).

In summary, the literature concurs that multiple obstacles exist to the use of formal
health services among indigenous and *mestizo* communities, including traditional belief
systems, cultural preferences, language barriers, the time and cost required for accessing
modern alternatives, and the poor quality of many of the available services. These findings
underscore the potential importance of the *Ley de Maternidad Gratuita and* PRO-AUS in
reducing the costs of modern treatment and ensuring the availability of medicines. However, they also underscore the importance of addressing staffing issues, to ensure adequate
clinic opening hours, and of radically improving the cultural sensitivity of services, especially those associated with childbirth. Involving traditional midwives in institutionalized
birth procedures is the most obvious way to overcome the cultural issues associated with
indigenous women's reluctance to use such services. Finally, the literature reveals a generalized distrust of, and reluctance to seek help from, outsiders. This suggests the importance
of training community volunteers to provide nutritional counseling for pregnant women
and for young children, and to promote IMCI protocols which can counteract damaging
superstitions related to the management of diarrheas and other childhood illnesses.

Rural Sanitation. Many rural families in Ecuador have deficient access to potable
water and sanitary services: 23 percent lack access to safe drinking water and 41 percent
lack access to safe sanitary services (MSP/INEC 2005). The available evidence suggests that
this remains a major factor underlying the incidence of digestive tract disease, since hygiene
practices are not adapted to this situation and there is widespread ignorance regarding

water supply quality and the dangers of untreated water. A study in the highland farming community of Tunshi-San Nicholas (Chimborazo province) found that food is not adequately washed, and water is not boiled because people (wrongly) believe it is treated. Utensils and areas used to prepare food are littered with remains of food and garbage and insects are omnipresent. People do not wash their hands before eating, even after agricultural work in which they work with animals or use agrochemicals (Harari and others 2000). This underscores the importance of incorporating water and sanitation interventions into the national nutritional strategy.

CHAPTER 4

Issues Facing Ecuador's Nutrition Programs

T his chapter reviews nutrition-related programs in Ecuador, compares spending levels and outcomes in similar countries, and presents an analysis of the coverage, cost per beneficiary, benefit incidence, and targeting efficiency.

Review of the Main Nutrition-related Programs in Ecuador

Coverage of and Access to Primary Health Care Programs

Nutrition strategy needs to be grounded in the primary health care system, because nutrition outcomes are determined, above all, by the interaction of feeding practices with the incidence and management of illness. This section surveys the aspects of the primary health system in Ecuador that are most pertinent to nutritional outcomes, and comments on recent developments, strengths, and weaknesses.

The health network of the Ministry of Public Health (*Ministerio de Salud Pública*, MSP) in Ecuador comprises 1,715 facilities, of which 72 percent are subcenters, the main point of entry of the primary attention network. The system is staffed by just under 31,000 professionals, of whom 18 percent are doctors, 11 percent are professional nurses, 21 percent are auxiliary nurses, and 40 percent are technical auxiliaries, or administrative or service staff (Table 24). Over the last decade, there has been little change in the scope of the network or the number of staff. However, in 2004, following an industrial dispute, doctors' working hours were halved, from eight to four hours per day. No compensatory increase in the number of doctors has been made, implying the risk of a significant reduction in the system's capacity. The MSP's service production statistics indicate that there has been a modest but steady increase in the production of most services in the last decade, in absolute terms and per

Table 24. Health Ministry Staff and Facilities, 1996–2004

	1996	1997	1998	1999	2000	2001	2002	2003	2004
Doctors	4,490	4,730	4,770	4,925	4,766	5,030	5,297	5,468	5,725
Dentists	1,046	1,097	1,107	1,193	1,234	1,269	1,375	1,398	1,416
Chemists	80	82	91	108	107	108	110	113	127
Obstetricians	624	637	680	761	754	770	842	784	759
Professional nurses	2,654	2,750	2,965	3,112	3,092	2,943	3,347	3,301	3,435
Lab. technicians	696	721	732	816	796	831	856	1,070	987
Auxiliary nurses	6,475	6,797	6,612	6,363	6,316	6,132	6,349	6,122	6,447
Others[a]	10,444	10,947	11,028	10,978	10,568	10,232	11,147	10,621	11,863
Total staff	**26,509**	**27,761**	**27,985**	**28,256**	**27,633**	**27,315**	**29,323**	**28,877**	**30,759**
Hospitals	120	124	122	121	121	121	118	114	126
Health centers	93	98	96	103	103	105	110	119	122
Subcenters	1,188	1,190	1,201	1,202	1,215	1,207	1,186	1,137	1,229
Health posts	241	240	238	236	223	229	238	230	238
Total facilities[b]	**1,642**	**1,652**	**1,657**	**1,662**	**1,662**	**1,662**	**1,652**	**1,600**	**1,715**

[a] Includes technical auxiliaries, administrative, and service staff.
[b] Excludes dispensaries.
Source: MSP.

capita of the population (Table 25). However, during 2002–04 there was a worrisome reduction in the number of medical consultations per 1,000 population, from 861 to 781, which might reflect the effect of reduced doctors' working hours. There was a strong increase in the coverage of prenatal consultations by the MSP during 1996–2004—from 61 percent to 82 percent. This trend was paralleled by the coverage of postnatal consultations,

Table 25. Health Ministry Service Production, 1996–2004 (per 1,000 population)

	1996	1997	1998	1999	2000	2001	2002	2004
Normal births	9	8	8	10	10	10	10	10
C-sections, abortions	2	3	4	4	4	4	5	6
Other surgery	8	6	7	8	8	8	9	9
Hospital discharges	24	22	24	24	24	24	26	27
Medical consultations	682	621	723	680	746	789	861	781
Dental consultations	0	94	100	99	121	106	113	142
Food rations	255	221	233	216	204	210	213	208
Total of all activities	979	976	1,098	1,041	1,117	1,151	1,237	1,183
Memo item: Population, million	11.59	11.77	11.95	12.12	12.3	12.48	12.66	13.03

Source: World Bank based on MSP statistics and demographic indicators. No data are available for 2003.

Table 26. Coverage of Maternal and Child Consultations by Health Ministry Facilities

	1996	1997	1998	1999	2000	2001	2002	2004
Total consultations								
Prenatal	225,569	201,443	256,274	266,810	273,903	280,015	308,187	297,724
Births attended	102,887	96,154	99,347	115,567	117,608	119,330	131,467	131,615
First consultations (children < 1)	279,372	281,808	305,774	305,431	344,290	326,064	364,268	285,752
Consultations as a % of pregnancies								
Prenatal consultations	61%	55%	69%	71%	74%	75%	83%	82%
Births attended	28%	26%	27%	31%	32%	32%	35%	36%
First consultations <1	76%	76%	83%	81%	93%	88%	98%	79%

Source: World Bank based on MSP statistics and demographic projections.

which rose from 76 percent to 98 percent during 1996–2002, before dipping to 82 percent in 2004 (Table 26).[20]

The 2005 Ministry of Health budget was $482 million, equivalent to 1.5 percent of GDP (Table 27), a fivefold increase since 2000. As seen above, this is not linked to a major increase in service production; rather, it reflects, in the main, the recovery of salaries in real terms, following their dramatic erosion during the 1997–99 inflation.

Ecuador's health and nutrition spending stands at about PPP$100 per capita. This is relatively low in absolute terms, but is broadly in line with what would be expected, given the level of Ecuador's GDP, compared with the rest of Latin America and with similar countries worldwide (Figure 20).

This suggests that—while it is important to maintain health and nutrition spending at least at the current level—it is also necessary to recognize that there is limited fiscal space for large increases in spending. For this reason, it is important to analyze the interprogrammatic distribution of funds and to ensure that the resources are optimally assigned, in terms of national priorities for improved health and nutrition outcomes. Equity criteria should be part of this discussion, and there should be a strong focus on understanding the efficient cost of reaching desired outcomes.

At present, Ecuador's nutrition status is inferior to that of other countries with similar levels of per capita health and nutrition spending, such as Morocco, Nicaragua, and Thailand (Figure 21). A similar unfavorable comparison can be made within Latin America with Brazil and Colombia (not shown in the graph). The challenge, in short, is to turn this spending into better nutrition outcomes.

---

20. The figure of 98 percent for 2002 seems unrealistically high and probably reflects confusion in the data between first consultations and subsequent consultations.

Table 27. Public Health Ministry Budget, 2000–05[a]

	2000	2001	2002	2003	2004	2005
	US$ million (current)					
Staff	65	99	172	196	224	279
Other current expenditure	30	27	42	54	56	72
Investment and capital expenditure	9	62	45	60	91	131
Total	**103**	**189**	**259**	**310**	**371**	**482**
	Percentage of the Total					
Staff	63	52	66	63	60	58
Other current expenditure	29	15	16	17	15	15
Investment and capital expenditure	8	33	17	19	24	27
Total	**100**	**100**	**100**	**100**	**100**	**100**

[a] Executed budget for 2000–04 and projected expenditure for 2005.
Source: MEF/STFS

Free Maternity Law and PRO-AUS

The Free Maternity Law (*Ley de Maternidad Gratuita*, LMG) was enacted in 1999 to promote free access to primary health care for mothers and children under 5. This aimed to offset the possible negative effect of the introduction of a cost-recovery system in the mid-1990s on

Figure 20. Health and Nutrition Spending in Relation to GDP, Selected Countries

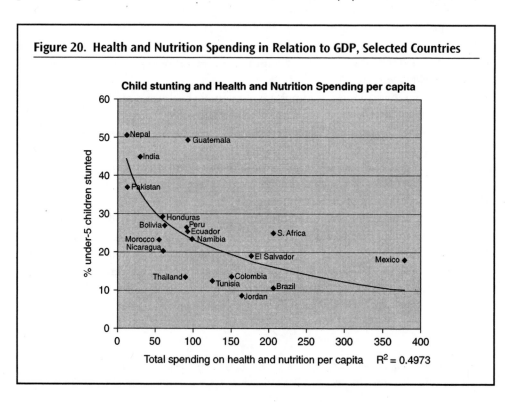

Figure 21. Child Stunting and Health and Nutrition Spending in Selected Countries

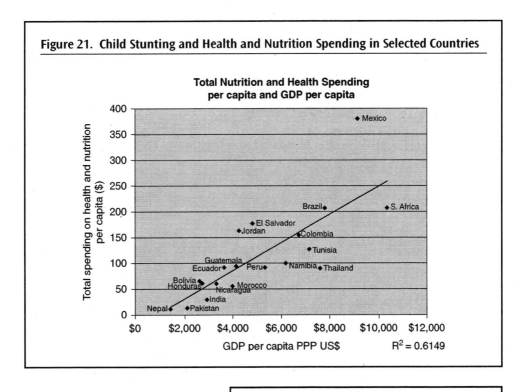

**Total Nutrition and Health Spending
per capita and GDP per capita**

$R^2 = 0.6149$

demand for these services. The LMG reimburses MSP health centers and hospitals on the basis of the estimated variable cost of the services they produce (excluding staff costs, which are provided through the core MSP budget). The LMG's executed budget in 2005 was $19.8 million, which represents about 4 percent of the total budget of the MSP.

The LMG has improved the supply of medicines in the public health system, including nutritional supplements (see Figure 22). However, the program has yet to advance significantly with plans to improve the cultural sensitivity of maternity-related services (for example, by allowing the remuneration of traditional midwives who bring their patients to institutional settings for

Figure 22. A Well-stocked Medicine Cabinet–Including Nutritional Supplements—Supplied by the LMG at the Alluriquín Rural Health Subcenter in Pichincha

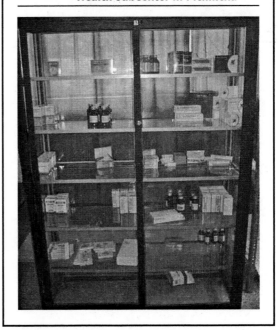

birth). Nor—due to budgetary constraints—has LMG been able to reimburse maternity-related services outside the MSP (for example, in the *Seguro Social Campesino*). It has also yet to complete the establishment of an adequate Management Information System that allows the tracking of service production and other relevant performance statistics.

The establishment of the PRO-AUS Universal Health Insurance System (administered by the *Secretaría de Objetivos del Milenio* [SODEM] and due to start operations by the end of 2006) will further strengthen the financing of basic health services for the poor in Ecuador. PRO-AUS will be limited to households in SELBEN Quintiles 1 and 2, paying for services not covered by the LMG. However, this also raises the need to coordinate efforts to finance basic health care for low-income families, in order to avoid unnecessary overlaps and to fully exploit managerial and administrative synergies.

Growth Monitoring—The SISVAN System

Monitoring of growth outcomes in Ecuador is the responsibility of the SISVAN system in the MSP. The system concentrates on the measurement of weight-for-age, which is recorded at health posts on a standard growth-monitoring chart. Each health post then remits summary statistics for the total number of cases measured and the proportion which is underweight, which are eventually processed into summary data at the national level.

In recent years there has been a worrisome decline in coverage of the SISVAN system (Figure 23). Having risen from 39 percent in 1996 to 74 percent in 1999, the proportion of pregnant women who are measured through SISVAN had declined to 33 percent by 2004.

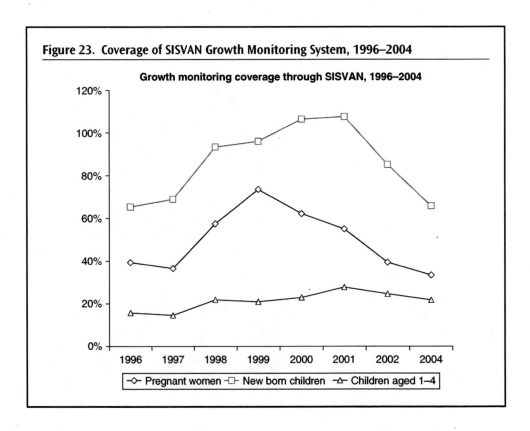

Figure 23. Coverage of SISVAN Growth Monitoring System, 1996–2004

Growth monitoring coverage through SISVAN, 1996–2004

Table 28. Coverage and Outcomes of Weight-for-Age Monitoring through the SISVAN System

	1996	1997	1998	1999	2000	2001	2002	2004
Coverage of weight-for-age monitoring (% of the relevant population)								
Pregnant women	39%	36%	57%	74%	62%	55%	39%	33%
(Children aged < 1)	65%	69%	93%	96%	106%	108%	85%	66%
Children aged 1–4	16%	15%	22%	21%	23%	28%	25%	22%
Proportion of cases measured which are reported as being underweight								
Pregnant women	24%	23%	25%	23%	27%	26%	25%	22%
New born children	n.d.	n.d.	n.d	n.d.	10%	13%	10%	10%
(Children aged < 1)	13%	11%	12%	11%	10%	11%	11%	12%
Children aged 1–4	24%	22%	21%	22%	20%	21%	21%	19%

Note: No data are available for 2003.

Source: World Bank calculation, based on SISVAN data and demographic indicators.

Similarly, according to official data, having purportedly risen from 65 percent to over 100 percent of the estimated number of births nationwide between 1996 and 1999, the registry of children under 1 year of age in the system slipped back to 66 percent in 2004. The weighing of children aged 1–4 has remained very low throughout this period. In all these categories, the proportion of those weighed who are deficient has remained stable through the period reviewed (Table 28).

In practice, few children are measured more than four times a year, and no mechanisms are in place to follow up on the measurement with effective counseling to improve weight gain. In addition, the broad, categorical approach of the data- reporting system means that no individual-level data are processed into the central registers (so that specific children cannot be tracked from month to month), and it is impossible to track deterioration within the range of "acceptable" or "unacceptable" weights, or to see what proportion of those measured is gaining weight adequately. And although children's height is often measured on their visit to a health post, these data are not processed by SISVAN (Figure 24).

The bands of the monitoring system are so broad that it is possible for a child to gain no weight at all for long periods, without this triggering any change of status. Figure 25 shows the chart for a child that grew normally in the first eight months of life, reaching 8.5 kg, but then grew only 1.5 kg (to 10 kg) in the following 14 months. Nevertheless, this child remains in the "green" zone of weight sufficiency. In a worst case scenario, a child could continue to weigh 11 kg between the ages of 9 and 30 months, but nevertheless remain in the category of normal weight.

SISVAN's emphasis on the "bands" of nutritional sufficiency—instead of the trajectory of the individual's growth—reflects an underlying confusion about the role of such charts. The primary function of growth charts is the diagnosis of individuals' needs as the basis for determining corrective actions, and not nutritional surveillance to assess the number or proportion of the population below certain cutoff points. For this reason, the Pan-American Health

Figure 24. Children's Height is Often Measured at the Health Post—But This Information is Not Processed in SISVAN

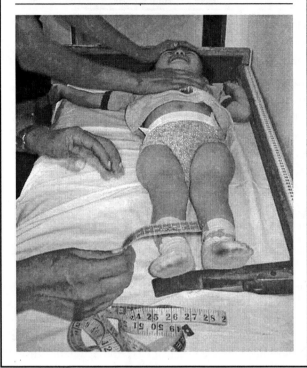

Organization (PAHO) is now encouraging countries to abandon the use of charts with colors and cutoff points and to focus on the trajectory of individuals' growth. PAHO also encourages plotting height-for-age in the health card, in addition to weight-for-age, as another key element of monitoring individual growth (personal communication, Dr. Chessa Luttter, PAHO).

Micronutrient Supplementation

During the past decade, the alleviation of micronutrient deficiencies has been given high priority in the nutrition programs of developing countries, because it has been shown to be highly cost-effective, and is relatively

Figure 25. A Child Growth Chart Illustrating a Typical Trend

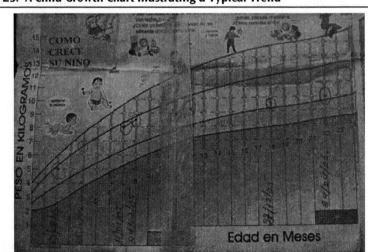

easy to manage. In 2004, micronutrient programs were ranked second among all possible development strategies, based on cost-benefit criteria by a panel of international economists, known as "The Copenhagen Consensus." This high rate of return arises from the large potential gains in labor productivity and the relatively low cost of these programs. Micronutrient malnutrition has linkages to six of the Millennium Development Goals: those pertaining to poverty alleviation; universal primary education; gender equality; reduced child mortality; improved maternal health; and the combating of HIV/AIDS, malaria, and other diseases.

One vital dimension of micronutrient strategy is the provision of supplements to key target groups. These are normally distributed through the primary health care system. Table 29 summarizes recommended interventions and their estimated costs, ranked by target group.

The role of the micronutrient program of the MSP has changed in recent years and needs to be clarified. Until 2003, it was responsible for distributing supplements in pill form, donated by UNICEF and other international agencies, through MSP health posts. However, such donations have stopped. The LMG provides funding for micronutrient supplements distributed in health posts, both regular and therapeutic dosages. In addition, the food distribution programs such as PANN2000, *Aliméntate Ecuador*, and INNFA (discussed below) include nontherapeutic dosages of basic micronutrients in the powdered food rations they distribute for mothers and children.

In this setting, there is no apparent role for the micronutrient office of the MSP in the distribution of supplements. Its role should now become one of regulation, monitoring, and supervision of the provision and use of supplements by other programs rather than that of direct agent. Its budget needs to be made sufficient to carry out that role adequately. One issue that should be discussed with the LMG is the advisability of moving toward the use of a "sprinkles" presentation, which combines the administration of the supplement with the ingestion of a normal diet.

Another important micronutrient issue pinpointed in the recent literature is the importance of delaying umbilical clamping, in order to maximize the transfer of iron-rich blood to the newborn child. It has been estimated that a three-minute delay in clamping (with the baby held below the placenta) can permit the transfer of sufficient additional iron to support two months' normal growth. Since a child does not receive iron through breast milk and must rely on the store in their body at birth until complementary feeding begins after 6 months of age, this is a critical potential gain (Chaparro and others 2006:1997–2004).

The second basic element of micronutrient strategy is the mandatory fortification of mass-consumption foods. The elements of a well-designed system include: legislation regulating food fortification for nationally produced and imported foods; technical regulations for fortification based on international (Codex Alimentarius–FAO) and/or regional (MERCOSUR) standards; the enforcement of standards with penalties specified in health codes and legal instruments; and quality control checks at the border, retail, and household level. Table 30 summarizes international standards and estimated costs for cereal fortification. Table 31 summarizes wheat fortification standards that have been adopted in a range of countries, including Ecuador.[21]

---

21. The Ecuador standard for vitamin B2 is considerably higher than the international standard or that actually used in most countries.

Table 29. Recommended Micronutrient Interventions and Indicative Costs, by Priority Intervention and Target Groups[a]

Interventions in priority order:	Target groups in priority order				
	I Under 2s	II Pregnant Women	III Adolescent Girls	IV Preschool Children	V All Population
I	For 9–24m: 6 - monthly vitamin A supplements. Cost per child/year = $0.03	Daily iron folate supplements, from second trimester. Cost per pregnancy = $0.55 – 3.17	Weekly Iron folate supplements Cost per year = $0.11	6-monthly vitamin A Supplements for children aged 24–59 months Cost per child/year = $0.03	Iodized Salt Cost per person/year = $0.20–0.50
II	Sprinkles mix for home–based fortification; 60 sachets per year Cost per child/year = $0.88[b]			Daily fortification of community-prepared food supplement Cost per child/year = $0.07	Fortification of sugar, wheat flour, or other staple foods. Cost per person/year = $0.30 (wheat); $0.68–0.09 (sugar)
III	For 6–24 mo: Zinc supplements during diarrhea Cost per child/year = $0.16			Zinc supplementation during diarrhea Cost per child/year = $0.16	Vitamin A fortification of cooking oil Cost per person/year = $0.07

[a] The costs cited in this table do not include distribution costs.
[b] Sprinkles can only be used starting at 6 months as they need to be mixed with food. The cost estimate reported in the table is based on Sprinkles' distributors' claims. However, Sprinkles' real costs in some countries in Latin America have been higher. For example, in Guyana the cost of 60 sachets is reported as US$2.70, plus costs of distribution (transport, health worker time, and so forth). The experience in Bolivia has been similar.
Source: Personal communication, Dr. Chessa Lutter, PAHO.

In Ecuador, the fortification of wheat flour dates from 1995, and was formalized through a ministerial resolution in 1996 which requires iron fortification (55 parts per million), folic acid (0.6 parts), tiamin (4 parts), niacide (40 parts), and riboflavin (7 parts). The iron currently being used (since 1996) is micronized reduced iron powder. However, this formulation provides only about half the bioavailability of ferrous sulphate, which is the preferred form of iron in modern fortification programs. A change of the norm is being considered but no decision has been taken.

The largest 22 flour mills, which account for 95 percent of the national market, are covered by the system. Imports are covered by the rules, but verification in customs is

Table 30. Cereal Fortification: Recommended International Standards

Nutrient	RDA* Units mg/day	EAR**	Chemical Sources Used in Cereal Fortification	Activity or Concentration %	Amount of Source to Supply 100% of RDA per kg ppm or mg/kg	Cost (2003 estimates with added processing factor)	
						$/kg active component	$ per 100,000 RDA
Iron	8.18	10.3,	Elemental Reduced Iron	97	10.3	2.2	2.2
	10#	13.2	Electrolytic Reduced Iron	98	10.2	2.8–7.1	2.8–7.1
			Ferrous Sulfate	32	31	4.9	4.9
			Ferrous Fumarate	32	31	11.1	11.1
			Sodium Iron EDTA	13.5	74	78.6	78.6
Zinc	11.8	3.6, 2.6	Zinc Oxide	80	12.5	2.3	2.3
	10#		Zinc Sulfate	36	28	13	13
Calcium	1000	855	Calcium Sulfate	23	4350	0.60	60
			Calcium Carbonate	40	2500	0.62	62
Selenium	0.055	.028, .021	Sodium Selenate	42	0.13	52	0.3
Iodine	0.15	0.095	Calcium Iodate	62	0.24	34	0.4
Folate	0.4	0.32	Folic acid	87	0.46	36	1.4
Vitamin B$_1$	1.2	1.0, 0.9	Thiamin Mononitrate	103	1.2	17	2.0
			Thiamin Hydrochloride	100	1.2	18	2.2
Vitamin B$_2$	1.3	1.1, 0.9	Riboflavin	100	1.3	28	3.6
Niacin	16, 14,	12, 11	Niacin (Nicotinic Acid)	100	15	7	11
	15#		Niacinamide	100	15	7	11

(continued)

Table 30. Cereal Fortification: Recommended International Standards (*Continued*)

Nutrient	RDA* Units mg/day	EAR**	Chemical Sources Used in Cereal Fortification	Activity or Concen-tration %	Amount of Source to Supply 100% of RDA per kg ppm or mg/kg	Cost (2003 estimates with added processing factor)	
						$/kg active component	$ per 100,000 RDA
Vitamin B₆	1.3	1.1	Pyridozine Hydrochloride	83	1.6	44	5.7
Vitamin B₁₂	0.0024	0.002	Cyanocobalamine, 1%	1	0.24	15,200	3.6
Vitamin A	0.9 or 3000 IU	0.42 or 1390 IU	Vitamin A Palmitate, 250 SD	250 IU/mg	12		42
Vitamin D	0.005 or 200 IU	0.005 or 200 IU	Vitamin D3, 100 SD	100 IU/mg	2		8
Vitamin C	90, 75, 75#	54,44	Ascorbic Acid	100	75	8.7	65

* Recommended Dietary Allowances (RDA) of the Food and Nutrition Board of the U.S. Institute of Medicine, 2001.
** Estimated Average Requirement from RNIs of FAO/WHO. If two numbers shown for RDA, first is for males, second is for females. Both RDA and EAR values for females are for non-pregnant, non-lactating adults (19–50 years).
# RDA used for cost calculation purposes.

Table 31. International Comparison of Wheat Fortification Standards (per 2003)

Country	Type* of Program	Vit B1 ppm	Vit B2 ppm	Folic Acid ppm	Niacin ppm	Zinc ppm	Iron/Type** ppm	Ca g/kg
Argentina	M	6.3	1.3	2.2	13		30-FS	
Australia	M[a]	6.4						
Azerbaijan	V	3.3	2.8	1.5	18	25	55-E	
Bahrain	M			1.5			60	(2.1)
Bangladesh	P	6.4	4.0	1.5	53	33	66-E	
Belize	M	4.0	2.5	1.5	45		60	
Bolivia	M	4.45	2.65	1.5	35.6		60	
Brazil	P,M			1.5			42	
Canada	M	6.4	4.0	1.5	53		44	(1.1)
Chile	M	6.3	1.3	2.2	13		30	
Colombia	M	6.0	4.0	1.54	55		44	
Costa Rica	M	5.4	3.6	1.8	45		45-FF	
Cuba	M	7.0	7.0	2.5	70		45	
Dominican Republic	V	6.0	4.0	1.5	55		60	
Ecuador	M	4.0	7.0	0.6	40		55	

*P = Proposed, V = Voluntary, M = Mandatory, R = Required for specific regions or states, LA = Level Added, otherwise value gives minimum level standard required in fortified flour.
** Iron types specified under regulations: FS = Ferrous Sulfate, E = Electrolytic reduced iron, FF = Ferrous Fumarate, R = Reduced iron.

undermined by contraband. The *Instituto de Ciencia y Tecnología* (ICT) is the agency within the MSP responsible for the operation of the system. The protocol for the control and monitoring program includes three to four visits per year to each mill, where a check is made of the availability on site of the required fortifying agent. The volume of purchases of fortifying agent is checked against total production volume and there is an eight-monthly chemical test in each plant, using photospectrometry of atomic absorption. The samples are coded and sent to the *Universidad Central del Ecuador* (in Quito) for blind testing. The program's approach to compliance is focused on advisory rather than punitive strategies. However, it operates in an irregular fashion due to the lack of budget in the ICT, which has only two staff in Quito and one field person per province. The 2005 budget for the program was US$18,000 and this was reduced in 2006 to US$10,000. The estimated cost for the full operation of the program is US$25,000. No impact evaluation has been carried out for this program; it is estimated that this would cost US$120,000.

These arrangements fall well short of recommended international standards for the regulation of compliance, which specify that quality assurance in the case of fortified products should cover the premix, industrial production, sites of further processing (for example, bakeries), retail outlets, and imported commodities. The process of quality assurance should involve regular checks by the food companies themselves coupled with periodic product checks by laboratories associated with government food safety and regulation organizations. The food industry itself is normally responsible for: regular checking of feed rates on fortification feeders (once per eight-hour shift), regular iron spot tests on flour (once per eight-hour shift),[22] and regular checking of premix usage against production levels (monthly). The government food regulation lab should be responsible for quantitative testing of iron on a weekly or monthly basis, and the quantitative testing of all added micronutrients on a monthly or quarterly basis. Government labs also can undertake less expensive qualitative tests such as the black light test for riboflavin and a similar test for vitamin A to assess whether (but not at what level) these micronutrients have been added.

International experience suggests that the adoption of national standards and legislation is seldom sufficient to assure full industry compliance. In some countries, quality assurance has become part of a larger agenda of public-private collaboration, which sometimes includes subsidies to offset the increased costs of fortified products. In India, private sector compliance has been increased by pressure from independent consumer organizations (in some cases assisted by international agencies). These organizations, sometimes equipped with state-of-the-art laboratories, routinely test products and then make their findings available to the news media.

Feeding Programs

Ecuador supports half-a-dozen food distribution programs of different sorts. These include:

- The School Feeding Program (*Programa de Alimentación Escolar*, PAE) administered through the Education Ministry and aimed at children aged 5 and up, enrolled in rural and urban-marginal public schools. PAE provides breakfasts and lunches which are prepared at the school with the help of parent volunteers.
- Several programs administered or financed by the Social Welfare Ministry (*Ministerio de Bienestar Social*). These include: (a) *Aliméntate Ecuador*, aimed at children 2–5 years of age whose families are in SELBEN Q1 and Q2; it distributes powdered reinforced food, ordinary food rations given as an incentive to take up by mothers, and de-worming pills; (b) *Operación Rescate Infantíl* (ORI), which supplies three full means a day to under-5 children in community-based crèches, and also pays teams of mothers to care for the children and prepare the food; (c) transfers to the *Instituto Nacional del Niño y la Familia* (INNFA), which supports similar community-level agencies; (d) the FODI program (formerly *Nuestros Niños*), which is mainly an early childhood development program delivered through NGOs, but some of whose modalities include feeding.

---

22. The iron spot test is used to check whether flour has been properly fortified. This is a simple, inexpensive procedure that should be run on fortified flour on a regular basis.

▓ The PANN2000 program administered by the MPH, which provides fortified powdered food and drinks to pregnant and nursing mothers and to children aged 6–24 months who attend public health centers and subcenters.

Integrated Food and Nutrition System and the New Food Security Law

Three of the above-mentioned programs (AE, PAE, and PANN2000) are grouped in the Integrated Food and Nutrition System (*Sistema Integrado de Alimentación y Nutrición*, SIAN), which was established on an ad hoc basis in 2003 and was formalized by an Executive Decree issued in late 2005. SIAN aims to rationalize the feeding programs, to promote more rigorous targeting and impact evaluations, and to articulate feeding interventions with the primary health network and with nutrition outcomes. For this reason, it is led by the MPH. SIAN has worked to systematize the scope of interventions by the different programs, eliminating most of the overlaps by age group. It has also discussed options to consolidate their budgets, in order to facilitate channeling more resources to the most effective interventions (such as those for children under 24 months of age).

It is not clear what was the rationale for including some programs in SIAN while excluding others, with similar goals, and also operated by the MBS (such as ORI, *Nuestros Niños*/FODI, and transfers to INNFA). However, it is noteworthy that the three programs included in SIAN are those which are administered in liaison with the World Food Program (WFP), which carries out the necessary acquisitions and handles the distribution of the products.

In early 2006, a new Food Security Law was passed. Since this is primary legislation, it supersedes the Executive Decree creating SIAN. At the time of writing, the implementing regulations for the new law had yet to be published. However, it is clear that, although the new law recognizes the existence of SIAN, it has created confusion about its future role. In particular, the new law specifies that the budget of the PAE should not be consolidated with those of PANN2000 and AE, as had originally been planned.

This development makes it urgent to redefine the role of SIAN. In doing so, this study suggests that the Government should consider refocusing SIAN to become the focal point for a national nutrition strategy, as an integral part of Ecuador's primary health care program, while leaving food policy leadership to the agriculture sector. The main emphasis should be on developing community-level growth promotion programs in high-risk areas, linked to effective outcome monitoring. It is questionable whether the School Feeding Program, PAE, should remain within this framework, since it is not targeted on an age group relevant to nutritional outcomes and its main goal is to provide an incentive to educational participation, not to have an impact on health or nutrition.

SIAN has recently focused on establishing mechanisms to "pass on" individually identified beneficiaries between complementary feeding programs which address different age ranges (AE, PAE, PANN2000). This should be rethought, since programs focused on children over two years of age are unlikely to have much nutritional impact and probably do not belong in the nutrition sector. Rather, SIAN should focus on promoting interventions which are likely to make a difference in stunting outcomes, and should take a lead in addressing the sector's weak internal institutionality. There is a tendency to make politically motivated staff appointments, and frequent leadership changes make it difficult for a clear long-term strategy to coalesce. To overcome this problem, Ecuador needs to develop a corps of technically competent nutrition program managers who are insulated from political interference. Stronger monitoring and impact evaluation activities for nutrition programs, led by STFS (as specified in the Executive Decree creating SIAN) would help to catalyze a transformation toward professionally managed programs with clear goals and stable strategies.

Human Development Grant

The Social Welfare Ministry (MBS) also supports the *Bono de Desarrollo Humano* (BDH), a cash transfer program which is targeted on the poorest 44 percent of families in Ecuador, using a proxy means test (SELBEN). Almost a million mothers are eligible for this program, receiving $15 a month, making this the most costly, by far, of the nutrition-related programs outside the main MSP program. The BDH is currently being revamped to turn it into a conditioned program, linking the transfer to participation in basic health and education programs.

Given the importance of behavior-related causes of malnutrition in Ecuador, as documented in Chapter 3 of this study, the shift of the BDH toward an emphasis on human development and on encouraging appropriate primary health and nutrition behaviors opens up an important opportunity for nutrition strategy in Ecuador. Recent studies in Colombia, Mexico, and Nicaragua have found that CCT programs—when coupled with appropriate supply-side interventions—can have an important impact on child growth outcomes. It will also be important to rationalize the conditions applied under related programs (for instance, PANN2000 also requires attendance at primary health care clinics, just as PAE requires attendance at school).

Spending on Nutrition-related Programs

Excluding the mainstream primary health budget, spending on nutrition-related programs reached US$251 million in 2005—roughly 0.9 percent of GDP (Table 32). The *Bono de Desarrollo Humano* (BDH) accounts for almost 70 percent of the total. In real terms, spending on these programs has been stable in the last three years. However, there is considerable instability in the budgeting process, reflected in the big fluctuations in spending by individual programs (especially PAE and PANN2000). There are also considerable divergences between executed expenditure and the original budget (executed spending ranged in 2005 from 68 percent of the budget for *Aliméntate Ecuador* [PRADEC] to 104 percent for ORI). This budgetary instability is, in itself, a significant factor undermining program effectiveness and merits priority attention.

Much of the problem is rooted in the financing of programs from special funds which require discretionary assignment. The food distribution programs are mainly funded from the special oil-related fund, CEREPs (not from normal fiscal resources). CEREPS transfers are discretionary and are often unpredictable and irregular. This leads to delays in the first part of the year, so that programs must juggle reserves held over from the previous year to keep their operations afloat. Inevitably, this leads to instability in service delivery. It also

Table 32. Expenditure Trends on Main Nutrition-related Programs, 2003–05

		2003	2004	2005
Executed Budget (current $mn)				
Bono de Desarrollo Humano	BDH	161.8	173.4	167.7
Prog de Alimentación de Niños y Niñas	PANN	5.7	3.5	9.8
Alimentate Ecuador (formerly PRADEC)	AE	7.0	8.1	10.9
Programa de Alimenación Escolar	PAE	14.3	26.9	15.1
Maternidad Gratuita	MG	19.8	20.1	19.9
Oganización de Rescate Infantíl	ORI	14.7	20.1	27.9
Nuestros Niños/FODI	FODI	13.8	10.8	n.d.
Total (formerly FODI)		**223.2**	**252.0**	**251.3**
Executed Budget in Constant 2003 $mn				
Bono de Desarrollo Humano	BDH	161.8	166.4	157.3
Prog de Alimentación de Niños y Niñas	PANN	5.7	3.4	9.2
Alimentate Ecuador (formerly PRADEC)	AE	7.0	7.8	10.2
Programa de Alimenación Escolar	PAE	14.3	25.8	14.2
Maternidad Gratuita	MG	19.8	19.2	18.7
Oganización de Rescate Infantíl	ORI	14.7	19.3	26.2
Nuestros Niños/FODI	FODI	13.8	10.3	n.d.
Total (formerly FODI)		**223.2**	**241.8**	**235.7**
Executed Expenditure as a % of Original Budget				
Bono de Desarrollo Humano	BDH	80%	86%	85%
Prog de Alimentación de Niños y Niñas	PANN	396%	233%	98%
Alimentate Ecuador (formerly PRADEC)	AE	57%	51%	68%
Programa de Alimenación Escolar	PAE	46%	88%	100%
Maternidad Gratuita	MG	105%	101%	100%
Oganización de Rescate Infantíl	ORI	58%	68%	104%
Nuestros Niños/FODI	FODI	96%	127%	n.d.
Total (formerly FODI)		**77%**	**84%**	**97%**
Executed Expenditure as % of Transfers Received in the Year				
Bono de Desarrollo Humano	BDH	100%	100%	100%
Prog de Alimentación de Niños y Niñas	PANN	100%	28%	114%
Alimentate Ecuador (formerly PRADEC)	AE	100%	108%	136%
Programa de Alimenación Escolar	PAE	94%	96%	169%
Maternidad Gratuita	MG	108%	101%	118%
Oganización de Rescate Infantíl	ORI	96%	87%	100%
Nuestros Niños/FODI	FODI	87%	99%	n.d.
Total (formerly FODI)		**100%**	**95%**	**106%**

Source: MEF/STFS. No data are available for the INNFA programs related to nutrition.

Table 33. Cost per Beneficiary and Overhead Margin for Nutrition-related Programs, 2005

	Cost per Beneficiary (US$/year)[a]	Adminis-trative Margin (%)
School meals (PAE)	12	11.5
PANN2000	51	12.2
Mi papilla	42	12.3
Mi bebida	62	12.1
BDH	205	12.2
Aliméntate Ecuador	22	22.7
INNFA	57	n.d.
Nuestros Niños	247	n.d.
ORI	534	11.1
Total		12.2%

[a] Including administrative overhead.
Source: World Bank calculations based on data from MEF/STFS and programs.

leads to major divergences between the amounts of money transferred to the programs and the accrued spending reported in the budget liquidation for any given year. In 2005, for example, PAE managed to spend an amount equivalent to 170 percent of the amount it received in transfers—while in 2004, PANN2000 spent only 28 percent. These complex, opaque arrangements, in which financial and physical reserves are held over between fiscal years, undermine transparency and accountability in the sector.

Table 33 shows program overhead costs and cost per beneficiary for the main nutrition-related programs. There are striking differences between the cost per beneficiary, which ranges from $12 a year for the School Feeding Program, PAE, up to the enormous sum of $534 a year for the Child Rescue Program (*Operación Rescate Infantil*, ORI) run by the Social Welfare Ministry (*Ministerio de Bienestar Social*).

These diverse amounts reflect the differences in benefits assigned by the programs—ranging from two or three distributions a year of a relatively small-value *papilla* (bag of powdered food) by PANN2000 and *Aliméntate Ecuador*, to a monthly cash-equivalent payment of $15 in the case of BDH to a full regime of three freshly cooked meals a day all year, in the case of ORI.[23] Nevertheless, there are also differences in value-for-money. PAE manages to deliver two meals a day for about 40 days a year for $13 per beneficiary—one-fortieth of the per beneficiary cost of ORI. Nevertheless, according to program data, the meals delivered

---

23. PANN2000 is also working to strengthen its nutrition education component, but this remains a small proportion of program costs.

by PAE contain 50 percent of the daily caloric requirement, 75 percent of the protein requirement, and 90 percent of micronutrient requirements. One of the big differences is that PAE uses unpaid volunteer labor from families to cook the food, while over a third of ORI's budget is spent paying and feeding mothers who care for the children and cook the food (Figure 26).

Declared overhead margins—the central administrative cost of the programs—are generally at reasonable levels, averaging 12.2 percent. The notable exception is *Aliméntate Ecuador*, whose very high margin of 23 percent reflects a mismatch between the size of the program's organization and the amount of budget resources it was able to mobilize in 2005. To reach an efficient margin given its present organizational dimensions, the program would need at least double the funds it was assigned in that year. However, most of PAE's overhead is buried in other parts of the Ministry of Education's budget. Similarly, PANN2000 draws on MPH staff time, not budgeted under the program (Figure 27).

A household that participates in more than one program can greatly increase the total amount of benefit it receives. The 2005 ENEMDU data set permits analysis of the overlap between the AE, BDH, INNFA, ORI, PAE, and PANN programs at the household level. These data is summarized in Table 34.

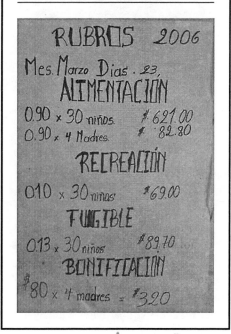

Figure 26. A Wall Chart at the *Semitas de Aliso* ORI Group in Cotopaxi Illustrates the Program's Costs, a Total of $50 per Child/Month—35 Percent of which Benefits the Mothers

Based on their survey responses, 67 percent of Ecuadorian households receive no support from any of these programs; 21 percent receive support from at least one program, 9 percent from two programs, 3 percent from three programs, and 1 percent from four programs. The average value of the benefit for those with one program was $109 per year; this rose to $182 for two programs, $229 for three, $380 for four, and $602 for the very small number of households benefiting from five programs. The overall national average for the benefit received per household/year from all these programs is $49.

Accountability at the Program Level

There have been strong efforts to improve the transparency and accountability of nutrition-related programs in recent years. This has included the adoption of new Management Information Systems (MIS) by AE, INFFA, ORI, and PAE. There are also efforts underway to coordinate across programs: many early childhood development programs in Ecuador

Figure 27. A Young Mother Collects the PANN2000 *Mi papilla* for Her Child at the Rural Health Subcenter at Alluriquín, Pichincha

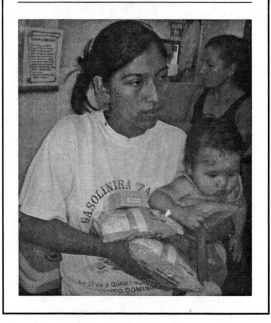

(including FODI, INNFA, ORI, and Pronepe) are using the *Matraca* information system. Several programs are also adopting modern quality management systems (AE, ORI, PAE). In contrast, other programs are still working to put their MIS in place (LMG). To improve transparency in procurement, several of the feeding programs have turned to PMA as a contracting agency (AE, PAE, PANN2000).

There have also been advances in the implementation of methodologically rigorous impact evaluations (AE, BDH, and PANN2000).[24] However, other programs (such as PAE) have begun impact evaluations which do not meet generally recognized standards for design and quality. STFS should assume a stronger role in the definition and supervision of impact evaluation strategies and should also work with programs to ensure that their monitoring and evaluation systems provide adequate information about program outputs and performance to permit effective goal-based management.

Program Coverage, Targeting, and Benefit Incidence

This section presents the results of an analysis of program coverage and benefit incidence, based on institutional data and on the December 2005 ENDEMU labor force survey. This survey—which has a large nationally representative sample of over 15,000 households—included questions designed to identify participation in the main social programs, including the main feeding programs.

---

24. The difficulties of implementing such studies are illustrated by the evaluation of PANN2000, carried out by PAHO. This study was designed longitudinally to follow children 6–12 months of age for 11 months, to coincide with their peak linear growth velocity, which is the period when an effect of the program on linear growth would be most likely to be observed. However, there was a three-month delay in program implementation, which reduced the exposure of the "intervention" group to the program from 12 to 9 months, likely reducing the impact measured by the study (Personal communication, Dr. Chessa Lutter, PAHO). On the other hand, the delivery of fortified complementary food to the "intervention" group in the study was considerably more frequent than has since been the norm across program beneficiaries since the study was undertaken, which would tend to result in an overstatement of program impact in the study.

Table 34. Overlap between Nutrition-related Programs at Household Level

No of Programs Received	No of House-holds[a]	% of House-holds	Average amount, US$/yr[b]	Total Value US$	Main Permutations observed[c]
0	2,124,840	67	0	0	
1	652,644	21	109	71,312,814	BDH, PAE, PANN, AE, ORI, INNFA
2	290,932	9	182	52,949,131	BDH+PAE, BDH+PANN, PANN+PAE, BDH+AE
3	89,328	3	229	20,472,777	BDH+AE+PAE, BDG+PANN+PAE
4	21,896	1	380	8,321,005	BDH+AE+ PANN+PAE
5	2,609	0	602	1,571,787	BDH+AE+ORI+PANN+PAE
Total	3,182,249	100	49	154,627,514	

[a] Covers AE, BDH, INNFA, ORI, PAE, and PANN. The total number of households and total program cost implicit in this table are lower than those generated by program data, due to underreporting of program participation, which is normal in survey-based data.
[b] Based on program data for cost per beneficiary. The estimate assumes only one beneficiary per program/household, so it is a lower bound.
[c] There are many more permutations, but they have very low incidences and contribute little to the weighted averages.
Source: World Bank calculations based on ENEMDU 2005. Number of observations: 18,537.

Table 35 shows the coverage of the target population for each program. These data were generated based on program data for the number of beneficiaries. The ENEMDU data set was used to estimate the size of the target population policy of each program. The school feeding program reports that it reaches 1.2 million beneficiaries—many more than it ought to, based on the declared beneficiary target population of rural and urban-marginal school children, who total of 922,000, a difference of 31 percent. It would make sense for this program to narrow its targeting, since it also has had a problem providing a full protocol of services. In 2005, it managed to provide only 43 days of service a year on average (based on the program's declared cost per beneficiary of $0.30 per day and the executed budget of US$15.7 million), against the target of 160 days a year for full service. In

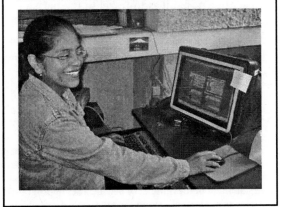

Figure 28. The MIS Officer at ORI's Regional Operations Center for Cotopaxi in Latacunga using the "Matraca" Information System

Table 35. Beneficiaries and Coverage Rates of the Main Nutrition-related Programs in Ecuador

	Beneficiaries	Target Population	Coverage	Definition of Target Population
PAE	1,303,857	922,229	141%	Children enrolled at school aged 5–14 in rural and urban-marginal areas
PANN2000				
Mi papilla	104,933	338,627	31%	Children aged 6–23 months
Mi bebida	86,769	n.d.	n.d.	Pregnant women
BDH	917,037	930,003	98%	Women under 65 in Q1 and Q2
Alim.Ecuador	247,886	358,598	69%	Children aged 2–5 in Q1 and q2
INNFA	60,774	1,503,815	4%	Children under 6
Nuestros Niños	17,249	731,780	2%	Poor children under 6
ORI	55,271	731,780	8%	Poor children under 6
Total	**2,697,223**			

Note: The beneficiaries for INNFA and *Nuestros Niños* registered in this table are those who receive food, and not those getting other types of service from those programs. See text for explanation of methodology.

Source: World Bank calculation. Data for beneficiaries from programs. Data for target population are based on ENDEMU December 2005.

an effort to correct this problem, PAE is developing a Geographic Information System with data on school location, which should provide the basis for better logistics and more consistent service delivery.

Other programs have a relatively high coverage level, for example, *Aliméntate Ecuador* with 69 percent, *Mi Papilla* with 31 percent, and BDH with 98 percent. In the case of AE, unfortunately, benefits are very small and the resulting nutritional impact is questionable. In AE, beneficiaries receive between two and three deliveries a year of a package of powdered food with micronutrient supplements together with antiparasite pills for children aged 2–5 whose parents are on the SELBEN Q1 and Q2 listings. They are also given standard food (including rice and cooking oil); the latter—which are added in order to increase the incentive of families to travel to the parish center to collect the products—make up more than half the cost of the benefit. PANN2000 has a similar problem: it delivers fortified powdered food up to eight times a year to mothers who bring children over 6 months old to check-ups. Yet, most mothers only come two or three times a year, so once again, the nutritional impact of the benefit is not likely to be very great.[25]

At the other end of the spectrum from PAE are ORI and *Nuestros Niños* (now called FODI). These programs deliver very large benefits to a very small proportion of the

25. Since the feeding programs administer rations, not people, they often have unreliable data on the number of beneficiaries, and simply impute them from the number of rations distributed, dividing by the prescribed number of rations per beneficiary/year. In the case of PANN2000, this probably leads to an understatement of the number of beneficiaries in program data, since the real amount of rations given to each beneficiary is smaller than the program's design protocol supposes.

Table 36. Benefit Incidence of Nutrition-related Programs in Ecuador[a]

	Population Deciles from Poor (1) to Rich (10)[b]											Progressivity
	1	2	3	4	5	6	7	8	9	10	Total	
Program	% of resources received by each decile											Index[c]
School meals (PAE)	23.8	19.8	13.4	12.7	9.6	7.6	5.8	3.9	2.3	1.1	100	0.40
PANN 2000	15.9	13.5	13.4	13.2	12.8	9.9	8.8	7.0	3.4	2.2	100	0.24
BDH	16.2	17.3	15.9	14.6	13.1	9.8	7.1	3.9	1.6	0.5	100	0.34
Aliméntate Ecuador	20.5	23.7	11.5	11.5	10.9	9.3	3.6	4.5	3.7	0.6	100	0.38
INNFA	14.0	10.5	13.3	19.6	10.2	11.9	8.3	3.6	5.8	2.9	100	0.21
ORI	28.3	19.0	14.3	7.5	14.1	5.5	3.8	3.5	3.8	0.3	100	0.43
Total	**18.0**	**17.6**	**15.3**	**13.6**	**12.8**	**9.1**	**6.7**	**4.1**	**2.1**	**0.7**	**100**	**0.33**

[a] Based on 2005 program data for costs and 2005 labor force survey for beneficiaries. Costs include program overheads.
[b] National population deciles based on income data from December 2005 labor force survey.
[c] This index number is so defined that a perfectly equal distribution (each population decile getting 10 percent of the program's resources) returns a value of zero. If all resources go to decile 1 (poorest), the index number takes the value 1 (maximum progressivity); if all resources go to decile 10 (least poor), it takes the value -1 (maximum regressivity).
Source: World Bank calculation from program data for costs and ENEMDU data for program participation and income.

potential target population (less than 10 percent in each case). This leads to serious problems of horizontal inequity (that is, other children in similar conditions do not get the same benefit). The administrative procedures of ORI are also open to abuse at the community level. Large amounts of cash are transferred to community committees on a per capita basis for the children enrolled in their programs, and this is used to buy food for preparation by mothers employed in the local community. This sets up an incentive to produce fraudulent lists of children in order to get more cash. The program has worked hard to establish audit mechanisms and administrative procedures to control this risk, but it is difficult to overcome.

Based on the ENEMDU data set coupled with administrative data for program costs, a benefit incidence analysis was conducted of the main nutrition-related programs. Responses to program participation questions were tabulated against the population decile (of per capita incomes) to which each household belongs, to determine what proportion of program resources is given to each decile. The results of this analysis are reported in Table 36, and the cumulative distribution of the resource assignment is graphed in Figure 29.

The results of this analysis show that all the programs are progressive, in the sense that they deliver more resources to poor than to rich households. However, there are considerable differences in the degree of leakage of resources into the higher end of income distribution. The average progressivity index number across the programs is 0.33. This index number is so defined that a totally flat distribution would report a value of 0, a fully regressive

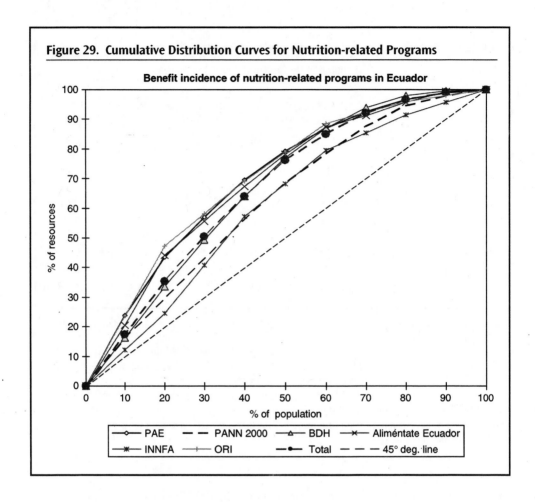

Figure 29. Cumulative Distribution Curves for Nutrition-related Programs

distribution (where all funds go to the richest decile) would give a value of –1, and a fully progressive distribution (with all funds going to decile 1) would give a value of 1.

On this measure, ORI is the most progressive program (lowest leakage into the non-poor deciles), with an index number of 0.43; and the School Feeding Program, PAE, also reports a relatively high score (0.40). *Aliméntate Ecuador* and BDH—which both use SELBEN as the basis for their targeting—have index numbers of 0.38 and 0.34, respectively. PANN2000 and INNFA have 0.24 and 0.21, respectively. However, a progressive benefit incidence should be considered a necessary, but not sufficient, condition for a social program. It is also necessary to ensure wide coverage (small errors of exclusion). This is particularly important when the benefits have a high value, as in the case of ORI and BDH.

There is also an issue about the choice of appropriate targeting mechanisms. In an effort to fight politicization and strengthen transparency, feeding programs have been adopting improved targeting procedures. For example, *Aliméntate Ecuador* has adopted the SELBEN proxy means test system, which identifies the bottom two quintiles of income distribution. This is a good system (albeit with a relatively high cutoff point) for programs whose principal aim is a general boost to families' economic conditions (such as BDH).

Box 11. School Feeding—The International Experience

School health and nutrition programs are normally concerned with educational impacts, rather than nutrition impacts. Accordingly, most studies relating to school feeding have examined the effect of these activities on school attendance, drop-out rates, and educational attainment, and the evidence points to the positive effect of such indicators (Del Rosso 1999). However, the effect of school feeding programs on nutritional outcomes is more controversial.

School-aged children have nutritional needs that can be addressed through such programs. Extra chores and long walks to school increase energy needs (Del Rosso 1999). Furthermore, intestinal worms, ranked first among the causes of disease in school-aged children, are common throughout the developing world. According to WHO estimates, more than 400 million children are infected worldwide (WFP).

School breakfasts are likely to have the most positive impact. A 2005 study of the impact of breakfast eating on nutritional adequacy, body weight, and academic performance found that while breakfast eaters consume more calories daily, they are less likely to be overweight. Consuming a morning meal may also "improve cognitive function related to memory, grade and school attendance" (Adams and others 2005).

However, school feeding programs may be badly targeted due to perverse selection. Malnourished or sick children are likely to start school later or not to attend school at all. A Nepal study found the probability of stunted and better-nourished children attending school was much lower (Moock and Leslie 1986). In Ghana, malnourished children entered school later than their well-nourished counterparts and completed fewer years of school overall (Glewwe and Jacoby 1994).

Lessons Learned

An international review of 18 school nutrition and health programs recommended the following as elements of "best practice":

- Target disadvantaged areas; in some countries it is appropriate to target girls.
- Ensure regular delivery.
- Assure community participation in planning and implementation.
- Include de-worming and micronutrient supplements (iron, folate, vitamin A, as needed).
- Make nutrition education a key component. This has a threefold potential value: take home messages for the family, messages to improve future reproductive health and parenting, and messages aimed at the improved health and nutritional status of these children at present.
- Coordinate among sectors (health, education, agriculture Ministries, NGOs).
- Optimize the timing of school feeding and the amount of food provided. Food delivered early in the day will improve the learning potential of children who did not receive breakfast at home. It may be best to provide a snack that is not seen as a meal replacement.
- Avoid disrupting the educational process: distribute food before or after school hours, and do not turn schoolrooms into kitchens during school hours.
- Be cost-efficient and avoid "capture" by suppliers. School feeding costs vary widely by country, depending on the size of the meal or snack, the number of students, food prices, and logistics of delivery. However, on standardized measures there appear to be very wide variations that almost certainly reflect inefficient procurement and capture by producers in some programs. One survey of Latin American school feeding programs found that costs per thousand kilocalories varied from $0.03 (Peru) to $0.84 (Paraguay).

However, given that malnutrition is more concentrated than poverty in Ecuador (the proportion in poverty is about double the proportion of children who are stunted and affects only slightly over 20 percent of children), it is questionable whether SELBEN is the best way to target nutrition programs. It would be better to target such programs on the communities where the problem of stunting is concentrated. However, care should be taken to avoid targeting at the household level based on the condition of individual children, due to the risk of perverse incentives.

CHAPTER 5

Recommendations for the Development of a Goal-based National Nutrition Strategy

The last three years have witnessed significant efforts to improve programmatic coordination in the nutrition sector, through the establishment of the *Sistema Integral de Alimentación y Nutrición* (SIAN), under the aegis of the Ministry of Public Health (MSP). However, SIAN now needs to develop a goal-based national nutrition strategy, which should not be limited to feeding programs but should take in all relevant interventions, including community-level growth monitoring and counseling, primary health, and micronutrient supplementation. SIAN should also coordinate with the agencies responsible for water and sanitation.

Define a Clear Goal

The strategy should start from a clear definition of the problem and setting of a goal. The problem on which Ecuador should center its attention is stunting. Ecuador has a stunting rate of 23 percent of the population under 5 years of age, which, in round numbers, is 300,000 children. It has adopted the goal of halving chronic malnutrition between 1999 and 2015, implying a target of 12 percent. In concrete terms, taking account of population growth, this would mean reducing the number of stunted children to 229,000 by 2010, and 183,000 by 2015. This implies tripling the rate of reduction of stunting, from 2 percent a year to around 6 percent. *This has been done by other countries and it is feasible for Ecuador today* (see Box 12 and Figure 30).

Strengthen Transparency and Accountability

The strategy should be anchored in a national nutrition monitoring system which is an effective instrument for orienting policy and holding programs accountable, nationally and

Box 12. Nutrition Success Stories

Ecuador faces a great challenge. To meet its target to halve malnutrition by 2015, it needs to triple the rate of reduction of stunting, to over 5 percent a year. But other countries have shown this can be done.

Thailand

Thailand reduced under-5 malnutrition (weight-for-age deficiency) from 25 percent in 1986 to 15 percent in 1995, and virtually eliminated protein-energy malnutrition. The key to this outcome was a strong consensus at the national and local levels about the priority of the intervention, including an understanding that this should be regarded as an investment, which permitted the use of foreign aid to complement domestic resources. Key features of program implementation were the use of community volunteers on a massive scale (1 per 10 households), coupled with a strong nutrition technical support organization. Thailand's success was centered on community-based growth monitoring promotion and health care efforts. This depended on high literacy levels plus village traditions of community service and group action. In contrast, community-based volunteerism in East African efforts documented by the International Fund for Agriculture Development (IFAD) were far less successful, with a 50 percent volunteer drop-out rate every two years.

Chile

Chile exhibited rapid and significant improvements in health and nutrition between 1965 and 1980. Growth retardation (under 75 percent of standard) dropped from 23.7 percent in 1965 to 1.9 percent in 1980 (Horwitz 1987). Today, only 1.7 percent of children are stunted in Chile. The integration of nutrition interventions and primary health care appears to have contributed most to these impressive outcomes. The provision of potable water and sewage control in urban areas also led to reductions in infant mortality (Horwitz 1987). Food supplementation (in the form of milk) benefited the poorest quintiles. Furthermore, "the country has perhaps one of the most sophisticated nutrition surveillance systems in the world. Data on approximately 400,000 children and 200,000 mothers are regularly collected, collated, analyzed, and used for decisionmaking by the Ministry of Health. There is a regular flow of information from every unit of the health system to the central computer service and back to each source, with appropriate comments when justified" (Horwitz 1987). Other factors in the success of this effort included: sustained political commitment, explicit attention to social equity, and outreach to isolated households and communities (mobile health units being more successful than stationary, often inaccessible, clinics).

Tanzania

Tanzania reduced child malnutrition (weight-for-age deficiency) from 50 percent underweight in the 1970s and early 1980s to roughly 30 percent by the early 1990s. The Joint Nutrition Support Program using UNICEF's "Triple A Cycle" process of community-based problem assessments and action plans established a pilot program in Iringa Province, which became Africa's showcase nutrition undertaking. Its dramatic success led to a rapid expansion through the 1980s and early 1990s to other areas of the country as the Child Survival and Development Program.

In the 1990s, however, nutrition outcomes stopped improving and infant and child mortality began increasing due to declining use of maternal and child health services in the country. This was due to the loss of focus on the issues of primary health and nutrition, as policy attention shifted to health sector reform with an emphasis on outputs and impacts. Inexplicably, community-based services (and nutrition) were excluded from this highly defined discourse (which covered service delivery only to the health facility level), and, in consequence, largely disappeared from the health sector agenda. The reform measures may even have contributed to worse primary outcomes, due to the inability of some low-income households to afford newly imposed user fees.

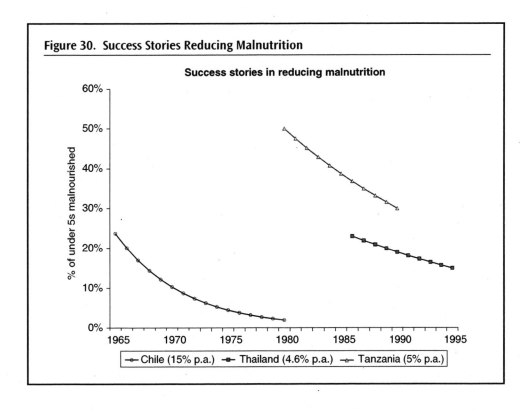

Figure 30. Success Stories Reducing Malnutrition

locally. The *Sistema de Vigilancia Alimentaria y Nutricional* (SISVAN) has deteriorated in recent years—it collects out-of-date data for only part of the problem (weight, not height) and for only part of the population and then does nothing with them. The current system confuses the monitoring of individual children (where what matters is growth trajectory in weight and length) with that of epidemiologic surveillance, which uses cutoff points to define the nutritional condition of a group. For surveillance purposes, a sampling methodology should be used that provides adequate desegregation and time points for planning purposes (for example, through family health surveys). In this context, the SISVAN system as such should be focused on providing information to inform immediate decisions about each individual child in vulnerable populations. Such decisions should be made locally, based on the growth pattern for weight-for-age, height-for-age (HAZ), and weight-for-height. To this end, SISVAN needs to be transformed using computerized techniques. The data should be used to supervise and guide local programs to achieve maximum effectiveness. But they should also be remitted to the central health system to facilitate follow-up when health areas are missing targets for the intensity of monitoring or are failing to follow up adequately on children whose growth trajectory is deficient. The system should also include height (or length) measurement and weight measurement, especially for children over 1 year of age. A key step to effectiveness—as seen in *Atención Integral a la Ninez-Comunitaria* (AIN-C)-type programs—is the sharing of information with mothers at the community level, to engage them in the process of the child's growth monitoring and help them correct the problems which cause stunting. Hand-held computers used by promoters may offer a workable option for combining effective feedback to mothers at the community level with the automatic generation of up-to-date registers of growth monitoring data for the use of health system managers. Over time, as the coverage and consistency of the data generated by SISVAN improve, the overall pattern of nutritional status reported by SISVAN should converge toward that reported in rigorous, survey-based epidemiological evaluations of nutritional variables.

SIAN should broadcast and monitor service-production standards and national and local nutrition outcome goals. Output targets should include the frequency of growth measurement and the coverage of basic protocols such as immunization and attendance at mother and child clinics. Outcome goals should include indicators for the proportion of children failing to grow adequately from month to month (intermediate indicators to be produced on a monthly basis), HAZ scores, and the proportion of children who are stunted (impact indicators). To make them meaningful, these goals should be calibrated, based on the starting point of each village.

Gear Program Configuration to the Distribution of the Problem

The programming of interventions should be adapted to the severity of the problem in different areas, giving high priority to communities with high-risk characteristics. In the *rural sierra*, which houses 40 percent of all stunted children, a full package of measures should be implemented, including community-based nutritional counseling and growth monitoring, improved health service access, nutritional supplements for pregnant mothers, appropriate complementary feeding for children over six months of age, water and sanitation investments, means-tested income transfers, and school feeding. In *other rural areas*, some of these interventions may not be necessary; decisions should be based on data about present circumstances. In *urban areas*, the emphasis should be placed on nutrition education and monitoring activities and means-tested income transfers. The distribution of food supplements to children over two years of age should be avoided in urban areas, due to the danger of producing overweight children.[26] *Nationwide*, nutrition education and micronutrient supplementation and fortification programs should be implemented.

Give High Priority to Community-based Growth Monitoring and Nutritional Counseling

International experience has shown that–much more than feeding programs–nutrition education and counseling programs at the community level are critical to achieving the behavioral changes needed to reverse Ecuador's poor nutrition outcomes. Such programs, which should constitute the keystone of the national strategy outlined above, are at present almost totally absent. Compared with the importance of establishing community-level mechanisms for growth monitoring and nutritional counseling, the debates about shifting resources between different complementary feeding programs such as AE, PAE, and PANN2000 are akin to rearranging the deck chairs on the Titanic.

---

26. This risk is likely to be minor in the case of PANN2000, which is focused on children under 2 years of are, and whose food rations supply only 30 percent of the estimated daily nutritional needs of the child. However, in programs focused on older children, the risk is greater. At present, the sporadic delivery of the *Aliméntate Ecuador Papilla* (for children aged 2–5) makes it unlikely that the program is contributing to obesity, but, given the lack of evidence of significant nutritional gains from the program, it is difficult to justify continuing to focus on this age range with this sort of intervention.

The Basic Support for Institutionalizing Child Survival (BASICS) project established such a model (*Atención Integral a las Enfermedades de la Primera Infancia* (AEPI) and registered marked successes in some parts of the country (such as Otávalo). However, when the project ended, the system was not effectively institutionalized. The growth monitoring system should be fully integrated within primary health care protocols and linked to the revival of a community-based approach to the Integrated Management of Childhood Illnesses (IMCI), such as diarrhea and respiratory illnesses, which was promoted heavily in the 1980s but has deteriorated over the last decade.

Rethink the Targeting of Nutrition Interventions

Ecuador's nutrition programs have worked hard to improve targeting in recent years and the benefit incidence analysis prepared for this report confirms that the outcomes are generally positive. Most programs now exhibit relatively low levels of leakage into the high end of income distribution. However, the degree of concentration among the poorest households in the bottom quintile remains patchy, and there is still too much leakage into non-poor populations in some programs (most notably INNFA and PANN2000). The findings of the benefit incidence analysis also raise some important issues about errors of inclusion and exclusion arising from the use of the proxy means test in SELBEN targeting, which should be addressed by the PPS in the forthcoming SELBEN 2 exercise.

Particularly noteworthy with regard to improved targeting is the strong action of *Aliméntate Ecuador* under the Palacios administration to end politicization and adopt a transparent targeting system, limiting eligibility to households which are certified as SELBEN Q1 and Q2. Similarly, PAE has worked to focus more strongly on poorer rural and urban-marginal communities, supported by a geographic targeting system developed with World Bank support. As a result, as shown by the benefit incidence analysis presented in this report, PAE is now one of Ecuador's most progressive social programs from a distributive standpoint, channeling 70 percent of its resources to households in the bottom two quintiles of income distribution.

Notwithstanding these improvements, the targeting procedures of Ecuador's nutrition programs still pay scant attention to the nutritional characteristics of the beneficiary populations, and too little emphasis is placed on the critical target groups (pregnant women and children aged under 24 months), where the right interventions could make a major difference to stunting outcomes over a relatively short time.

For this reason, the generalized tendency to use SELBEN Q1 and Q2 for targeting nutrition programs merits reconsideration. This is the right method to use to target income transfers, such as BDH, but leads to too-broad a scatter of resources for nutrition-specific interventions. This report recommends that the targeting of nutrition programs be based on the nutritional characteristics of the population, at the community (not individual) level.[27] The 300,000 stunted children under 5 years of age–who should be the main object of nutritional strategy–represent only 23 percent of the under-5 cohort. This is a good benchmark for determining the ideal target population for nutrition interventions.

---

27. Access to benefits should not be directly linked to the individual child's nutritional status due to the risk of creating perverse incentives.

Improve the Equity of Resource Distribution

It is difficult to compare cost-effectiveness of Ecuador's feeding programs, due to radical differences in program design and purposes. However, there are clear issues of inconsistent program design. Some programs distribute very small benefits, while others have very high benefits which are difficult to justify. These inconsistencies turn the feeding programs into something of a lottery for beneficiaries, some of whom receive very large benefits (such as three full meals a day, every day, under ORI), while others receive three or four packets of complementary food annually (as with AE). These differences are reflected in program costs. Some are very cheap, raising doubts about what they can reasonably hope to achieve. A case in point is *Aliméntate Ecuador*, with costs per beneficiary of US$22 per year, reflecting the erratic delivery of relatively small benefits and a high overhead margin. PAE (although cheaper at US$13 per beneficiary) delivers more substantial benefits, reflecting the cost–economy that comes from scale and from using volunteers at the community level, but they are still erratic. In the middle of the range are PANN2000 and INNFA which have costs per beneficiary of US$51 and US$57, respectively. At the other end of the range are BDH ($205) and ORI (with per capita costs of a huge $534 a year).

The existence of programs with such large benefits merits attention. BDH has a relatively broad scope–reaching nearly 1 million of the poorest households—and has a transparent targeting system (SELBEN). These factors help to justify the size of the benefit. In contrast, ORI reaches only 55,000 children. This is too small a proportion of the relevant population to justify such a large benefit, because too many others in similar conditions are excluded. Such errors of exclusion are an important–and sometimes overlooked–source of horizontal inequity. They are particularly important when–as in the case of ORI—access to the program is governed by opaque procedures, conditioned on the organization of community bodies, which must be certified by the program. This type of arrangement is prone to political manipulation. So, although ORI has relatively small errors of inclusion, it is difficult to justify the scale of the program's benefits.

Overall, it would make sense to rationalize the feeding programs to establish more consistent norms for the definition of the value of benefits and to prioritize models which achieve the best "bang for the buck" in terms of products delivered to clients, and which have transparent targeting rules. It is also important to achieve appropriate scale, in order to avoid large overheads. Some programs have very high overheads, reflecting a lack of balance between the dimensioning of their central organization and the size of the program (for example, *Aliméntate Ecuador*). The problem of duplicated distribution costs could probably be improved if programs were reorganized to minimize geographic overlaps. (However, it should also be noted that the delegation of distribution to PMA by AE, PAE, and PANN2000 allows some synergies to be achieved within the present institutional setting, through the contracting of the same company for all three programs' distributions in a given province).

Make Conditionality Consistent Among Programs and Ensure
it is Functionally Efficient

Several of the programs reviewed condition food or cash incentives on the take-up of relevant services, such as primary health care consultations (BDH, PANN2000) or school enrollment and attendance (BDH, PAE). There is a need to review the definition of over-lapping conditions, to ensure consistency. There is also a need to ensure that such conditions do not provoke inefficient increases in demand, which might lead to suboptimal allocations of the limited available supply-side resources.

For example, at present, the MSP's formal protocols require eight doctors' visits in the first year of life, and this is the condition that has been established in order to receive the PANN2000 complementary food packages, *Mi Papilla*. While this level of controls is ideal, it does not take account of the fact that the public health sector in Ecuador is severely resource constrained—a situation that was worsened by the reduction of the doctors' working day from eight to four hours, as was agreed following a strike in 2004. In rural health posts, many women who turn up are unable to get a *cupo* for a consultation on that day and are turned away (thus losing the corresponding *Mi Papilla*). Even worse, if the eighth visit for one child crowds out the first visit of another, that would be severely sub-optimal. To reduce the risk of such outcomes, it might be advisable to rethink the rules for benefit eligibility to link them to minimum, rather than ideal, levels of attendance at the health post. This should be complemented by establishing lower-cost, community-level growth monitoring and nutritional advisory services.

The introduction of conditionality linked to BDH poses a similar risk—that health posts might be swamped with mothers seeking simply to certify their eligibility for BDH, as has happened in the pilot phase of a similar program in Peru (JUNTOS). The BDH con-ditionality rules should be designed to avoid provoking health post visits for the sole pur-pose of certifying eligibility and should rely on information generated by the MSP. Similarly, although this is not a nutrition sector issue per se, the PAE program should adopt strict rules to avoid the disruption of the school day by activities linked to the preparation and consumption of food. At present, there is a tendency for classrooms to be taken over during teaching time for families to prepare the lunches which are cooked on-site.

Address Erratic Service Delivery by Consistent Budgetary Programming and Realistic Program Goals

One reason for ineffective service or benefit delivery is the irregular nature of budgetary transfers to many programs, leading to "on–off" patterns of service delivery (for example, AE, PAE, PANNN2000). In the first quarter of 2006, AE had so few resources available that the only places where it was actively distributing its product were the communities that had been sampled for the intervention group of its impact evaluation! Similarly, PANN2000 had reportedly exhausted its stocks of *Mi Papilla*.

Typically, no money is transferred to any of these programs in the first half of the year, so they must operate based on stocks and financial reserves held over from the previous year. Not only are these arrangements inadequate to avoid erratic service delivery, under-mining effectiveness, but they also undermine transparency, because creative accounting leads to a mismatch between reported expenditures and real service delivery in a given bud-get period. There is a clear need to regularize the budget transfers to nutrition programs.

The problem of erratic services is also due, in part, to the establishment of overly ambi-tious coverage goals which are not consistent with budget availability. As a result, PAE con-sistently fails to deliver meals for more than 45 days a year (much less than half the school days) in large sectors of the country. As argued above, it would be better to narrow the targeting, to ensure that the populations most vulnerable to nutritional failure get a full service, while avoiding the dissipation of effort through broadly cast but thinly spread programs, which have little impact and are vulnerable to politicization.

A further dimension of the problem of erratic service delivery is the use of PMA for procurement. While this arrangement guarantees transparency, it also leads to a considerable, inflexible three-month lag between the availability of funds and the delivery of services at the community level, compounding the impact of erratic budgetary flows. This is due to PMA's requirement that the funds be placed in its bank account before procurement can begin. The Government should explore options to overcome this—perhaps by agreeing to framework contracts with suppliers, which can be instantly activated when funds become available.

Strengthen the Micronutrient Supplementation and Fortification Systems

One area where policy needs great strengthening is micronutrients. A critical element of micronutrient strategy is the mandatory fortification of mass-consumption foods. Ecuador was a leading country in Latin America in the development of food supplementation norms for the salt and wheat industries: salt iodization has been implemented since the 1980s, and the fortification of wheat flour dates from 1995. But the country has fallen behind the curve by failing to update its norms to take account of technological developments (for example, in the specification of the required iron supplement), and the micronized iron currently being used has little beneficiary effect. It also needs to greatly strengthen the system for monitoring compliance. Ecuador should consider outsourcing much of this activity to universities.

A second dimension of this issue is the distribution of appropriate micronutrient supplements to targeted populations (such as folic acid to pregnant women). In the past, the micronutrient program of the MoH distributed supplements donated by UNICEF, in tablet form. But the UNICEF donations have ended and LMG is now the source of funding for supplements (both regular and therapeutic dosages) distributed in health posts. The available evidence suggests that this has led to improvements in supply. The fortified food packages (such as those given by AE, INNFA, and PANN2000) also contain a nontherapeutic dosage of micronutrients. In this context of changes in financing and delivery arrangements for micronutrient supplements, Ecuador needs to redefine the role of key agencies. Rather than competing for a distribution role, the MoH's micronutrient program should focus on the regulation, monitoring, and supervision of the provision of micronutrient supplements by other agencies.

Appendixes

Ecuador Malnutrition Rates Using the New Reference Growth Charts

The New Reference Curves

Infant growth charts are used to monitor nutritional status and to assess child growth. In 1977, National Center for Health Statistics/Centers for Disease Control (NCHS/CDC) infant growth charts based on formula-fed infants, and at the time widely used in the United States, were subsequently adapted by the World Health Organization (WHO) as an international reference.[28] After a comprehensive review started in 1993, WHO concluded that the growth of breast-fed infants should be the norm, because breast milk is the ideal source of nutrition for infants. The main objective of the effort is to be able to properly target all grades of malnutrition to be able to have the most significant impact on improving child survival: about half of child mortality in developing countries is related to the effects of mild-to-moderate malnutrition as opposed to severe malnutrition (De Onis, Garza, and Habicht 2006).

---

28. The National Center for Health Statistics (NCHS) growth curves were constructed by combining two distinct data sets compiled in different time periods. For children under 2 years of age the data came from the Fels Longitudinal Study carried out in Yellow Springs, Ohio, from 1929 to 1975; the Fels curves reflect the growth of children who were fed primarily infant formula and in whom complementary feeding often was initiated before 4 months. The group was of homogeneous genetic, geographic, and socioeconomic backgrounds. For older children, the data came from nationally representative cross-sectional surveys of children in the United States and include all ethnic groups and social classes. Furthermore, the younger children were measured supine (length) and older children were measured standing (height). As a result there is a marked discrepancy in estimated height status immediately before and after 24 months of age, where the two curves ideally should merge seamlessly. This disjunction of about half a standard deviation or 1.8 cm, complicates the interpretation of growth data from nutrition surveys and surveillance activities. In addition, there is a positive skew in the weight distribution, reflecting a substantial level of childhood obesity. This upward skewness reflects an "unhealthy" characteristic of the NCHS reference population and may result in the misclassification of overweight children as "normal" (De Onis, Garza, and Habicht, 2006).

For this purpose, the WHO and the United Nations University, in collaboration with several research institutions, initiated the Multicentre Growth Reference Study (MGRS). The study developed a set of international growth charts for infants and children through 5 years of age based on the growth of healthy infants and children fed according to WHO recommendations (breast-fed at least 12 months and complementary food introduced sometime between 4 and 6 months) and living in healthy environments that do not limit their genetic growth potential. Moreover, the growth standards are based on a worldwide sample in recognition that environmental differences and not genetic endowment are the principal determinants of disparities in child growth.[29]

The new reference curves are expected to offer a single international standard that describes the best physiological growth for all children under 5 and to establish the growth of breast-fed infants as the normative model for growth and development.

Applying the New Reference Curves to Our Sample

We use the new reference curves to calculate malnutrition rates for our sample and to compare them with the previous results, obtained using the current growth curves.[30] Figure A.1 compares the distribution of the z-scores calculated using the new reference curves with the z-scores calculated using the current reference curves. There appears to be a clear shift of the height-for-age z-score distribution (an indicator of chronic malnutrition) to the left, signaling that chronic malnutrition is actually worse than estimated with the current curves. The curve for weight-for-age, or underweight, shifts slightly to the right, showing that underweight rates are somewhat overreported using the current charts. Finally, the new distribution of wasting (or weight-for-height), moves a little to the right, even if at the left tail it crosses the current distribution, causing an increase in the measured prevalence of acute malnutrition. For all weight-based indicators the shape of the WHO curves during infancy differs from that depicted by the NCHS, because the WHO standards are based on breast-fed infants (which have a different pattern of growth than formula babies). Thus, the results solve the critical problem of the NCHS inappropriateness for assessing growth of healthy breast-fed babies.

Table A.1 summarizes prevalence of malnutrition by area and socioeconomic characteristics comparing results obtained from the current and new reference curves.

Changes in prevalence vary by anthropometric indicator and age group. Overall stunting rates increase by about 6 percentage points, from 23.1 percent to about 30 percent, making the problem even more serious for Ecuador. On the other hand, underweight decreases by more than 3 percentage points. Both results are consistent with what is observed in other countries.[31] Note that stunting rates increase more significantly for the most vulnerable groups: around 10 percentage points higher for indigenous populations (the stunting rate is almost 55 percent!) and children of mothers with no education,

---

29. The MGRS collected primary growth data and related information from approximately 8,500 children from widely different ethnic backgrounds and cultural settings (Brazil, Ghana, India, Norway, Oman, and the United States). See de Onis and others (2001) for more details on the sample.

30. Calculations are done using WHO Anthro 2005, available for download on the WHO website.

31. Based on email correspondence with Mercedes De Onis, May 2006.

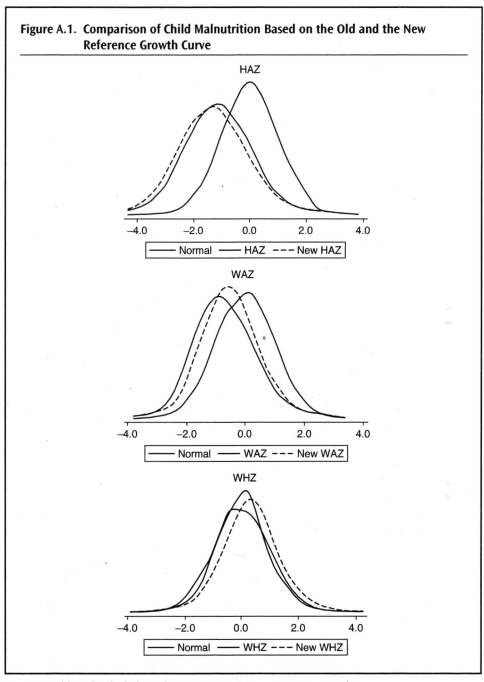

Figure A.1. Comparison of Child Malnutrition Based on the Old and the New Reference Growth Curve

Source: World Bank calculation using ENDEMAIN 2004 — CEPAR — Ecuador.

and about 7 percentage points higher for poor children living in rural area and in the Sierra region.

Multivariate analysis using the new reference curves shows results very similar to those found in previous sections (see Table A.1), the only difference being the way malnutrition increases for different age groups, as expected given the slightly different shape of the curve.

Table A.1. Comparison of Malnutrition Based on the Old and the New Reference Growth Curve

	Stunted (old)	Stunted (new)	Wasted (old)	Wasted (new)	Under-weight (old)	Under-weight (new)
Male	24.0	30.6	1.5	1.9	8.7	5.9
Female	22.0	27.1	1.5	2.1	9.6	5.5
Age						
0–5	3.3	8.1	1.5	6.4	0.5	3.2
6–11	9.5	12.1	2.5	3.8	6.4	3.5
12–23	28.3	31.5	4.1	3.5	12.8	6.4
24–35	24.6	38.3	0.8	0.9	12.2	7.1
36–47	27.4	33.7	0.0	0.0	9.9	7.3
48–60	27.9	29.9	0.5	0.5	6.9	4.2
Self-definition						
Indigenous	46.7	55.5	2.4	3.3	15.3	11.7
Mestizo	21.0	26.7	1.5	1.8	8.5	5.1
White	18.5	21.7	0.7	1.3	5.5	3.2
Black	14.3	21.6	0.6	2.8	11.2	6.7
Interviewer's Assessment						
Indigenous	45.5	54.3	2.4	3.4	15.5	11.5
Mestizo	21.4	27.1	1.4	1.9	8.6	5.2
White	9.2	11.2	3.6	2.0	2.0	0.0
Black	10.6	14.9	0.4	1.2	10.2	5.5
MEF's Education						
No education	38.7	48.2	0.3	2.2	17.4	7.6
Primary	29.9	37.2	1.5	2.2	11.2	7.5
Secondary	16.7	21.3	1.4	1.7	7.1	4.3
University	11.5	14.4	2.0	1.9	4.9	2.6
Number of Children<5						
One	19.5	24.7	1.5	1.3	7.8	4.3
Two	26.3	32.7	1.3	2.5	10.1	7.5
Three	27.7	34.9	2.1	3.3	11.6	6.2
Number of Women >14						
One	24.0	29.8	1.1	1.4	8.9	5.9
Two	21.2	26.4	1.5	2.6	10.9	6.3
Three	21.7	28.9	3.0	3.7	7.6	4.1

Table A.1. Comparison of Malnutrition Based on the Old and the New Reference Growth Curve *(Continued)*

	Stunted (old)	Stunted (new)	Wasted (old)	Wasted (new)	Under-weight (old)	Under-weight (new)
Area						
Urban	16.9	22.2	1.7	2.1	7.6	4.3
Rural	30.6	37.2	1.2	1.9	11.0	7.4
Region						
Sierra	31.8	38.2	1.3	1.5	10.2	6.4
Quito	29.9	34.0	1.0	1.3	8.4	5.1
Urbana	19.4	26.1	2.0	1.7	6.8	3.3
Rural	38.1	45.0	1.0	1.4	12.4	8.2
Costa	15.6	20.8	1.5	2.2	8.1	4.9
Guayaquil	11.8	15.6	1.2	2.3	6.7	4.4
Urbana	14.8	21.1	2.3	2.4	8.7	4.5
Rural	20.2	25.2	0.9	1.9	8.6	5.9
Amazonia	22.8	31.5	2.9	3.8	10.3	7.5
Insular	8.5	17.1	0.0	6.4	9.6	7.5
Consumption Quintiles						
Q1	30.0	36.5	1.5	2.3	12.1	7.7
Q2	24.3	30.3	1.7	2.0	8.9	6.0
Q3	17.3	24.1	1.0	1.8	7.1	3.9
Q4	18.6	23.6	0.6	1.3	7.3	4.2
Q5	11.3	13.5	2.9	2.5	5.2	3.4
Poor	27.6	33.8	1.6	2.1	10.7	7.0
Non-poor	16.4	21.7	1.3	1.8	6.8	3.9
Head of the HH						
Man	22.9	28.6	1.5	1.9	9.2	5.6
Woman	24.4	30.8	1.2	2.4	8.8	6.2
Altitud in Meters						
0–1,499 m.	16.6	21.9	1.6	2.4	8.3	5.1
1,500–2,499 m.	34.4	40.6	2.1	2.0	11.6	8.0
>2,499 m.	34.8	41.6	0.8	1.3	10.6	6.7
Total	**23.00**	**28.90**	**1.50**	**2.00**	**9.10**	**5.70**

Source: World Bank calculation using ENDEMAIN 2004—CEPAR—Ecuador.

Indicators

Anthropometric

Children

The World Health Organization (WHO) has long recommended the use of a reference population for the assessment of the nutritional status of children (Waterlow and others 1977; WHO 1979, 1983; WHO Working Group 1986). The International Reference Population advocated by the WHO was developed by the U.S. Centers for Disease Control (CDC) based on data from the National Center for Health Statistics (NCHS). The reference curves were obtained from two different populations.

For children below the age of 2 years, the sample is small and is based almost exclusively on white, middle-class children attending the FELS Research Institute in Ohio. The children's recumbent lengths were measured for the FELS data. For children aged 2 to adulthood, the WHO/NCHS/CDC cross-sectional curves are based on the relatively large and nationally representative sample of children obtained from the first National Health and Nutrition Examination Survey in the United States. Therefore, it also includes non-whites and children from low-income households. The children's standing heights were measured for the NCHS data (Hamill and others 1979).

In order to be able to compare the growth attainment of children of different ages by sex, the ENDEMAIN anthropometric measurements will be converted into three indexes: height-for-age, weight-for-age, and weight-for-height. Using the WHO/NCHS/CDC curves, the growth attainment of each child will be expressed as a standard deviation from the median (z-scores) (Waterlow and others 1977; WHO Working Group 1986). The z-score measures the degree to which a child's measurements deviate from what is expected

Table B.1. Cutoff Points for BMI, Adults

Classification	BMI Range
Underweight (Chronically Energy Deficient)	
Mild	17–18.49
Moderate	16–16.99
Severe	<16
Normal	18.5–24.99
Overweight	>=25
Pre-obese	25–29.99
Obese Class 1	30–34.99
Obese Class 2	35–39.99
Obese Class 3	>40

Source: WHO (1995, 2000).

for that child based on a reference population. The formula for the calculation of the height-for-age z-score is:

$$z_i = (Y_i^{s,a} - H^{s,a})/\sigma^{s,a}$$

where z_i = z-score for child i; $Y_{.i}^{s,a}$ = measured height (in cm) for child i of sex s and age a; $H^{s,a}$ = median height (in cm) for children of sex s and age a in the reference population; and $\sigma^{s,a}$ = standard deviation in height (in cm) for children of sex s and age a in the reference population.[32]

In the reference population, 2.3 percent of the children had a z-score less than −2, and 16 percent had a score of less than −1. These levels are generally expected for a "normal" population. We then calculated malnutrition rates as the percentage of children under 5 whose z-score was two standard deviations below the reference value. Children were defined as stunted if their height-for-age z-score was used, as wasted if their weight-for-height score was used, and underweight if their weight-for-age score was used.

Adults

The Body Mass Index (BMI)–weight in kilograms over height in meters squared–is the most common indicator of adult nutritional status.[33] BMI measures the thinness or obesity of adults controlling for the fact that weight is influenced by height and, therefore, is less biased by this relationship than other indexes. Moreover, by being correlated with fat mass, BMI is a good index of body energy. The WHO Expert Committee on Physical Growth suggests that a BMI of 18.5 should be seen as the minimum requirement for adequate health and proposes the classification presented in Table B.1.

---

32. For example, in computing the z-score for height-for-age of a 17-month-old boy, the child's height was compared to the distribution of height among 17-month-old boys in the international reference population (the median and standard deviation are 81.4 cm and 3.0 cm, respectively). If the index child is 76.5 cm tall, his height is 1.63 standard deviations below the median and he is assigned a z-score of −1.63.

33. BMI is an appropriate indicator for white individuals living in Europe or North America, but its appropriateness has been questioned for other populations that differ in body build and proportions (WHO Expert Committee 1995).

Table B.2. Prevalence Levels of Malnutrition among Adults

% of population with BMI <18.5	Classification
5–9%	Low Prevalence—warning signal, monitoring required
10–19%	Medium Prevalence—poor situation
20–39%	High Prevalence—serious situation
>40%	Very High Prevalence—critical situation

Source: WHO (1995).

Table B.2 shows the prevalence levels of adult malnutrition and specifies which levels would indicate the existence of a public health problem.

Micronutrients

Another important aspect of malnutrition is a lack of adequate micronutrients, that is, those minerals and vitamins needed by the body in small amounts for different functions that are essential to healthy growth and development. Micronutrient deficiency is an important cause of poor health, learning disabilities, blindness, and premature death. Generally, micronutrient deficiencies refer to inadequate amounts of iron, vitamin A, and iodine.

Iron is essential for the production of hemoglobin, which helps to deliver oxygen from the lungs to body tissues, to transport electrons in cells, and to synthesize iron enzymes that are required to use oxygen for the production of cellular energy. Vitamin A is an essential micronutrient for the normal functioning of the visual system, for growth and development, and for the maintenance of epithelial cellular integrity, the immune function, and reproduction. Iodine is required for the synthesis of thyroid hormones, which are involved in regulating the metabolic activities of all cells throughout the lifecycle. In addition, it plays a key role in cell replication. This is particularly relevant for the brain since neural cells multiply mainly in utero and during the first two years of life. Data on micronutrients were not collected in the ENDEMAIN survey, so our analysis draws mainly on the DANS survey (1986), the latest national nutrition survey, and on less representative studies.

Model and Methodology

This Appendix describes the methodology that we propose to use to study the main determinants of child malnutrition in Ecuador, to shed light on the relative importance of those individual, household, and community factors that are thought to influence stunting rates in the country (Chapter 3). We are particularly interested in disentangling the relationship between altitude, ethnicity, and child nutritional status.

Use of the Available Data

As discussed in Chapter 2, the main input to this analysis is the ENDEMAIN 2004[34] (Demographic and Mother and Child Health Survey). The survey consists of two related surveys: a household survey (10,985 households) and a mothers survey (10,814 women of fertile age).[35] The two samples are drawn from separate dwellings within the same censal segments. [36] The sample design allows inferences to be drawn at the national, urban, rural, regional, and (for the first time) provincial level.

---

34. The Bank has received the database and corresponding documentation.

35. Numbers refer to individuals (mothers and head of households) who have answered the complete questionnaire.

36. The original survey design proposed a single sample but the complexity of the instruments led to refusals to complete the interview during the pilot test; as a result the survey was divided into two elements. However, the fact that each survey was randomly sampled within the same (relatively small) censal segments allows the analyst to use the data sets together.

Table C.1. Observations by Type of Questionnaire

	Household Questionnaire	Women (MEF Questionnaire)	Children MEF (Questionnaire)
Short consumption module	7,315	8,147	18,669
Long consumption module	3,615	2,621	5,942
Weight	—	—	5,285
Height	—	—	5,286
Height-for-age z-score	—	—	5,214
Weight-for-height z-score	—	—	5,164
Weight-for-age z-score	—	—	5,216
Height above sea level[a]	—	—	24,206
Total[b]	10,985	10,814	24,696

[a] Data on height above sea level have been patched into the database using the GPS coordinates for sampling points provided by the survey firm coupled to map resources available within the Bank.
[b] The slight difference in the number of z-scores for analysis from the total observation of weight and height is due to the exclusion of outliers.
Source: Authors elaboration based on ENDEMAIN 2004.

Both surveys provide household expenditure data[37]; basic household demographics; and information on the characteristics of the dwelling, access to basic services, and participation in government programs. In addition, the household survey provides detailed data on household demographics and epidemiological characteristics, access to health services, and health spending (using a standard health demand survey format). The mothers' survey (using standard family health and epidemiology survey questions) collects details on fecundity, mortality, and mothers' knowledge, attitudes, and practices (KAP) related to reproductive health and maternal health KAP, as well as registering anthropometrics (weight and height) for the mother and for children under 60 months of age; and ethnicity of the mother.

The analysis of child malnutrition will be based on the "mothers" survey, using the household survey to complement information at the community level. Given the potential importance of altitude as a cause of nutritional outcomes, data on height above sea level have been patched into the database using the Geographic Information System coordinates for sampling points provided by the survey firm, coupled to map resources available within the Bank. Table C.1 provides an overview of the number of observations on expenditure, z-scores, and altitude available in the data set.

---

37. Two distinct instruments were used for registering expenditure: a short expenditure questionnaire, applied to 75 percent of households, and a detailed questionnaire, applied to 25 percent. Each of these formats was used in both of the surveys (households and women). Unfortunately, the resulting expenditure data sets are not directly compatible. This poses some difficulties for developing an instrumental variable for expenditure, for use in the econometric analysis; the team is exploring the options.

Modeling Child Health Determinants:
The Microeconomic Model of the Family

The theoretical model underpinning the econometric analysis is the basic microeconomic model of the family (Becker 1981; Singh, Squire, and Strauss 1986). The Beckerian microeconomic model of the family provides the basic theoretical framework for a number of empirical studies of determinants of nutritional status (Behrman and Deolalikar 1988). According to the simplified one-period model, households maximize the following utility function:

$$U = u(X, L, N),$$

where X and L represent the households' consumption of a composite good (the vector of consumption goods of different individuals in the household) and the household members' leisure, respectively, and N is the nutritional status of household members. Households maximize their utility function under several constraints, including a time constraint for each household member, a budget constraint for the entire household, and a biological nutrition production function:

$$N = n(I, Z, h).$$

The nutrition production function n relates the nutritional status of the child (the age and sex standardized anthropometric measure, either height-for-age or weight-for-age) to his or her past health status and the proximate determinants as outlined in the framework in Chapter 3. In this simplified one-period model, nutrition is a function of a set of inputs chosen by the household (including food intake, breast-feeding, use of health facilities, and the time dedicated by the mother to health-related activities), a set of exogenous characteristics (Z), which include the child's age and gender, the parents' health and education, and other household and community factors that influence a child's nutrition. η is a stochastic error term representing unobserved individual, household, and community characteristics affecting children's nutritional status.[38]

Ideally, one could estimate the effect of variables that directly influence a child's nutritional status by estimating the simultaneous system of the health production function and input demands. Unfortunately, the structure of the analysis is severely constrained by what data are available. The health production function is a complex relationship that cannot be captured easily by regression analysis based on cross-sectional survey data. It is best estimated with longitudinal data, which provide sufficient information to make it possible to make reliable judgments on the relative importance of different proximate determinants on growth attainment at the individual level.

The estimation of the health production function is further complicated by the fact that input use may be correlated with the error terms. The major source of bias arises from unobserved heterogeneity in the outcomes; in other words, the use of inputs is correlated with factors unknown to the researcher. For example, parents may take a child to the hospital more often if they are aware of the child's weak physical condition. In the face of such endogeneity, a model for the causes of health outcomes which included the use of health

---

38. For more details on the formulation of the health production function, see Behrman and Deolalikar (1988).

facilities as an independent variable and did not take into account the child's initial health endowment would underestimate the effects of the use of health facilities.

Researchers have often adopted instrumental variables and fixed-effects models to address this concern. Unfortunately, identifying instruments for inputs is often a difficult task. Moreover, it is almost impossible to measure all the inputs that enter into the health production function. Omitting inputs—or failing to calibrate for the quality of inputs—that are correlated with other included input (or instruments) could yield biased estimates.

Cluster fixed-effect models can be used to control for missing variables at the cluster level (in other words, at the family/household level). The main problem in using fixed-effect models is twofold: (a) if dummy variables are included for every fixed effect (such as for every family or every cluster), computation may not be feasible (in other words, if we added one dummy for each household); and (b) if the fixed effect is differenced away, then the effect of those variables that do not vary within a cluster (such as income in the household or infrastructure in a community) will be lost in the estimation process. Moreover, fixed effects do not work if nonlinearities are omitted in the model and if the unobservable variables affecting the health production function are not fixed.[39]

Reduced-form and Quasi-reduced-form Estimation

In the absence of adequate instrument and fixed-effect models, estimating reduced-form equations has proved to be a viable solution. Estimation of the reduced-form anthropometry function n does not provide information on the biological mechanisms responsible for children's growth deficits, but it does provide a consistent statistical framework within which to estimate the impact on children's health and nutrition of household and community exogenous variables that are generally open to policy intervention. The parameter estimates of the coefficients in the reduced-form equation can be interpreted as the *full* effects of exogenous covariates, that is, their effects not mediated by the proximate determinants.

The microeconomic model of the family can be solved to yield a reduced-form equation for health outcomes in which child anthropometry depends only on exogenous individual, household, and community characteristics:

$$N_i = n(C_i, C_h, C_c, \varepsilon_i),$$

where N_i is the height-for-age z-score for child i;

C_i are the individual characteristics of the child, including age and sex;

C_h are household characteristics that incorporate measures of family background, including resource availability, parents' health, and parents' skills measured generally by their level of education, and whether the father is absent from the household;

C_c are community characteristics, including the availability of health services, the state of infrastructure such as water and sewerage, food prices, and other community characteristics that affect child health through the proximate determinants; and

ε_i is an individual specific random disturbance associated with the anthropometric outcome of the indexed child and is assumed to be uncorrelated with the C variables.

---

39. Multilevel (random effects) linear models offer an alternative to fixed-effect models but do require additional assumptions about the distribution of the error terms.

An alternative to the simple reduced-form approach is to estimate a quasi-reduced-form model (Behrman and Deolalikar 1988; Sahn 1989), which differs from the standard model in that it includes some predicted inputs from the health production function (like consumption or quality of water or sanitation) and some variables from the reduced-form demand equation. Compared to the traditional reduced form, this approach has the advantage of controlling for the endogeneity bias and helping to explain the effect of some policy instruments, such as the availability of household resources. On the other hand, interpreting results from this kind of study is difficult, because they disclose niether the total effect of exogenous changes nor all of the structural parameters. We will estimate a quasi-reduced-form model in which per capita household consumption and program participation will be instrumented.

Instrumenting Per Capita Household Consumption

It is important to distinguish between exogenous and endogenous variables when investigating the determinants of child health. Exogenous variables, such as parent's education and height, are predetermined and have values that are not affected by the outcome of the process under examination (children's nutritional status, in this case). On the other hand, endogenous variables, such as the use of medical care and breast-feeding, are under the control of the parents and have values that are determined by forces operating within the model. For example, parents are more likely to bring their children to a medical provider if they think their children are sick. Including endogenous variables without further control would result in biased estimated coefficients.

Per capita household consumption is plausibly endogenous because it is likely to be affected by unobserved characteristics that also affect child nutritional status. Household resources, and particularly the component derived from mother's earnings, are likely to be endogenous because the consumption, leisure, and time allocation decisions are taken simultaneously with child health.[40] For example, women with more malnourished children tend to allocate more time to child care and less to work. The line of causation would therefore go not only from income to malnutrition but also from malnutrition to income. The simultaneity bias would affect the estimate of consumption and all the other variables that are correlated with income. In search for an instrument it is necessary to find variables that have good predictive power on consumption but that are not correlated with child health status. We use two identifying instruments to control for the endogeneity issue and for possible measurement errors: (a) a measure of durable household assets developed using categorical principal component analysis (Kolenikov and Angeles 2004), and (b) a dummy variable that reflects which consumption questionnaire was applied in the household. Consumption data are derived from a detailed expenditure questionnaire and a less detailed one, which are not comparable. Introducing the dummy allows us to combine the two data sets and also serves as an excellent instrument for consumption because it has good predictive power on consumption (by capturing the variability introduced by the different questionnaire used) and is not correlated with children's nutritional status (because the different questionnaires were randomly applied to households).

---

40. Following child health literature in which one assumes that the husband contributes no time to the production of child health (Horton 1986; Barrera 1990; Thomas, Strauss, and Henriques 1990).

Table C.2. Parameter Estimates of Reduced Form Models for Height-for-Age Z-score[a]

Model[b]	(1)	(2)
Log of consumption	0.27***	0.29***
	[0.07]	[0.08]
1 = 6–11 months	−0.57***	−0.58***
	[0.09]	[0.09]
12–23 months	−1.26***	−1.26***
	[0.08]	[0.08]
24–35 months	−1.13***	−1.13***
	[0.08]	[0.08]
36–47 months	−1.29***	−1.29***
	[0.08]	[0.08]
48–59 months	−1.31***	−1.32***
	[0.08]	[0.08]
Male	−0.17***	−0.16***
	[0.04]	[0.04]
HH size	−0.06***	−0.06***
	[0.02]	[0.02]
Number of children <5	−0.07**	−0.07**
	[0.04]	[0.04]
Number of women >14	0.15***	0.15***
	[0.03]	[0.03]
Men head of the HH	0.00	0.01
	[0.06]	[0.06]
Mother's age	0.06***	0.07***
	[0.02]	[0.02]
Mother's age sq.	−0.00***	−0.00***
	[0.00]	[0.00]
Mother's years of education	−0.05**	−0.05**
	[0.02]	[0.02]
Mother's years of education sq.	0.00**	0.00**
	[0.00]	[0.00]
Mother's height in meters	5.35***	5.25***
	[0.36]	[0.37]
Indigenous	−0.06	−0.03
	[0.10]	[0.10]
Urban	0.11**	0.17***
	[0.05]	[0.06]
Altitude in meters	−0.17***	−0.16***
	[0.02]	[0.02]

Table C.2. Parameter Estimates of Reduced Form Models for Height-for-Age Z-score[a] (Continued)

Model[b]	(1)	(2)
Knowledge	0.29***	0.28***
	[0.05]	[0.05]
Prop. of families with earth floor	—	−0.44**
	—	[0.20]
Prop. of families with toilet	—	0.29
	—	[0.18]
Prop. of fam. w/garbage collection	—	−0.21
	—	[0.16]
Prop. of fam. w/water from river	—	−0.02
	—	[0.08]
Prop. of families with fix tel.	—	−0.01
	—	[0.11]
Prop. of families with cellular	—	−0.13
	—	[0.14]
Prop. of families with TV	—	−0.34*
	—	[0.18]
Prop. of families with radio	—	0.16
	—	[0.16]
Constant	−10.45***	−10.34***
	[0.75]	[0.81]
Observations	2,688	2,687
R-squared	0.27	0.27

* Significant at 10 percent.
** Significant at 5 percent.
*** Significant at 1 percent.
[a] The dependent variable is expressed in standard deviations. Standard errors are in brackets.
[b] For model specification, see text.

In Chapter 3 we present the estimation results of four basic regression models (Table 7). The second model includes an innovative variable constructed to reflect the mother's expectations of her child's size (by comparing her opinion of her child's nutritional status at birth with objective data for its birth weight). Note that exact information on the child's birth weight is available for a large proportion of the children but not for all of them. For the children without exact birth weight data, mothers were simply asked whether the child had low weight at birth or not. We combined this information with the detailed birth weight information to construct the variable on expectation of child's size. In addition, we estimated the same models over a smaller sample of children, for which there is an exact estimate of the birth weight. The models are presented in Table C.2. As can be seen, the estimates are consistent with those from the larger sample.[41]

---

41. Similar results, not presented here, are obtained if we control for access to health centers, which is likely to be correlated to the exact estimates of birth weight.

Table C.3. Parameter Estimates of Reduced Form Models for HAZ with Different Definitions of Consumption

	Large Questionnaire			Short Questionnaire		
	Instrumented	Non-instrumented	Assets Index	Instrumented	Non-instrumented	Assets Index
Log of	0.19	0.02	—	0.36***	0.11***	—
consumption	[0.18]	[0.07]	—	[0.08]	[0.04]	—
Assets index	—	—	0.10	—	—	0.21***
	—	—	[0.10]	—	—	[0.05]
6–11 months	−1.10***	−1.10***	21.11***	−0.41***	−0.42***	−0.43***
	[0.17]	[0.17]	[0.17]	[0.09]	[0.09]	[0.09]
12–23 months	−1.43***	−1.44***	−1.43***	−1.27***	−1.29***	−1.29***
	[0.14]	[0.14]	[0.14]	[0.08]	[0.08]	[0.08]
24–35 months	−1.45***	−1.47***	−1.48***	−1.14***	−1.13***	−1.13***
	[0.14]	[0.14]	[0.14]	[0.08]	[0.08]	[0.08]
36–47 months	−1.70***	−1.73***	−1.72***	−1.26***	−1.27***	−1.27***
	[0.15]	[0.15]	[0.15]	[0.08]	[0.08]	[0.08]
48–59 months	−1.54***	−1.56***	−1.56***	−1.34***	−1.33***	−1.33***
	[0.15]	[0.15]	[0.15]	[0.08]	[0.08]	[0.08]
Male	−0.34***	−0.35***	−0.35***	−0.11***	−0.10***	−0.11***
	[0.08]	[0.08]	[0.08]	[0.04]	[0.04]	[0.04]
HH Size	−0.03	−0.04	−0.04	−0.07***	−0.08***	−0.09***
	[0.03]	[0.03]	[0.03]	[0.02]	[0.01]	[0.01]
Number of children <5	−0.11	−0.12*	−0.11*	−0.04	−0.06*	−0.05
	[0.07]	[0.07]	[0.07]	[0.03]	[0.03]	[0.03]
Number of women >14	0.21***	0.22***	0.20***	0.14***	0.15***	0.14***
	[0.07]	[0.07]	[0.07]	[0.03]	[0.03]	[0.03]
Men head of HH	0.05	0.06	0.05	0.01	0.01	-0.01
	[0.11]	[0.11]	[0.11]	[0.06]	[0.06]	[0.06]
Mother's age	0.04	0.03	0.03	0.08***	0.08***	0.08***
	[0.05]	[0.05]	[0.05]	[0.02]	[0.02]	[0.02]
Mother's age sq	0.00	0.00	0.00	−0.00***	−0.00***	−0.00***
	[0.00]	[0.00]	[0.00]	[0.00]	[0.00]	[0.00]
Mother's years of	0.00	0.00	0.00	−0.03	−0.03	−0.03
education	[0.04]	[0.04]	[0.04]	[0.02]	[0.02]	[0.02]
Mother's years of	0.00	0.00	0.00	0.00	0.00*	0.00*
education sq	[0.00]	[0.00]	[0.00]	[0.00]	[0.00]	[0.00]
Mother's height in	5.44***	5.61***	5.50***	5.62***	5.73***	5.66***
meters	[0.66]	[0.65]	[0.65]	[0.35]	[0.35]	[0.35]
Indigenous	−0.11	−0.17	−0.14	−0.12	−0.17*	−0.14
	[0.18]	[0.17]	[0.17]	[0.09]	[0.09]	[0.09]
Urban	0.47***	0.44***	0.45***	0.06	0.08	0.07
	[0.11]	[0.11]	[0.11]	[0.06]	[0.06]	[0.06]

Table C.3. Parameter Estimates of Reduced Form Models for HAZ with Different Definitions of Consumption (*Continued*)

	Large Questionnaire			Short Questionnaire		
	Instrumented	Non-instrumented	Assets Index	Instrumented	Non-instrumented	Assets Index
Altitude in meters	−0.16***	−0.16***	−0.17***	−0.18***	−0.17***	−0.18***
	[0.04]	[0.04]	[0.04]	[0.02]	[0.02]	[0.02]
Knowledge	0.18*	0.19**	0.20**	0.24***	0.26***	0.26***
	[0.10]	[0.10]	[0.10]	[0.05]	[0.05]	[0.05]
Prop. of families with earth floor	−0.66*	−0.65*	−0.62*	−0.08	−0.09	−0.05
	[0.34]	[0.34]	[0.34]	[0.18]	[0.18]	[0.18]
Prop. of families with earth toilet	−0.16	−0.12	−0.15	0.31*	0.31*	0.24
	[0.32]	[0.32]	[0.32]	[0.17]	[0.16]	[0.16]
Prop. of families w/garbage collection	−0.87***	−0.83***	−0.86***	0.03	0.08	0.03
	[0.32]	[0.31]	[0.31]	[0.16]	[0.15]	[0.16]
Prop. of families w/water from river	−0.29**	−0.30**	−0.28*	0.08	0.06	0.10
	[0.14]	[0.14]	[0.14]	[0.07]	[0.07]	[0.07]
Prop. of families with fix telephone	−0.25	−0.18	−0.24	0.11	0.21**	0.14
	[0.22]	[0.21]	[0.21]	[0.11]	[0.11]	[0.11]
Prop. of families with cellular	−0.07	0.01	−0.05	−0.13	−0.03	−0.08
	[0.25]	[0.24]	[0.24]	[0.13]	[0.13]	[0.13]
Prop. of families with TV	0.08	0.10	0.07	−0.44***	−0.42**	−0.47***
	[0.33]	[0.33]	[0.33]	[0.16]	[0.16]	[0.16]
Prop. of families with radio	0.18	0.28	0.29	0.04	0.09	0.08
	[0.33]	[0.31]	[0.30]	[0.15]	[0.15]	[0.15]
Constant	−8.84***	−7.98***	−7.48***	−11.84***	−10.39***	−9.20***
	[1.58]	[1.28]	[1.25]	[0.80]	[0.69]	[0.67]
Observations	855	857	856	2,790	2,791	2,795
R-squared	0.34	0.34	0.34	0.29	0.31	0.31

Standard errors in brackets.
* Significant at 10 percent.
** Significant at 5 percent.
*** Significant at 1 percent.

Models 1, 2, and 3 presented in Chapter 3 use an instrumental variable approach to the estimation of consumption, while model 4 uses, instead, an non-instrumented asset index. Here we present the results of the full regression models including consumption directly, without instrumenting it. Results are presented separately for the samples with the two different consumption questionnaires—the more detailed and the less detailed one. Table C.3 presents the estimation results comparing the models with instrumented and non-instrumented consumption and with asset index (non-instrumented). The coefficients' estimates are very stable across models and do not differ in size and magnitude from the estimates of the models using the combined sample presented in Chapter 3.

BIBLIOGRAPHY

ACC/SCN. 1992. "Second Report on the World Nutrition Situation." United Nations Administrative Committee on Coordination/Sub-Committee on Nutrition. Geneva.

Adams, Judi, Beverly L. Girard, Jordan Metzl, Mark A. Pereira, and Gail C. Rampersaud. 2005. "Breakfast Habits, Nutritional Status, Body Weight, and Academic Performance in Children and Adolescents." *Journal of the American Dietetic Association.* Chicago.

Albó, X. 2004. "Ethnic Identity and Politics in the Central Andes: The Cases of Bolivia, Ecuador, and Peru." In J. Burt and P. Mauceri, eds., *Politics in the Andes: Identity, Conflict, Reform.* Pittsburgh: University of Pittsburgh Press.

Alderman, H., and L. Christiaensen. 2004. "Child Malnutrition in Ethiopia: Can Maternal Knowledge Augment the Role of Income?" *Economic Development and Cultural Change* 52:287–312.

Alderman, Harold, J. G. M. (Hans) Hoogeveen, and Mariacristina Rossi. 2005. "Reducing Child Malnutrition in Tanzania—Combined Effects of Income Growth and Program Interventions." World Bank Policy Research Working Paper No. 3567. Washington, D.C.

Andrade, B., and C. Valle. 1981. "Breast Feeding: Causes for its Discontinuation in 2 Cities in Ecuador." *Boletín de la Oficina Sanitaria Panamericana* 91(5):408–17.

Araujo, C. 2005. "Iron Deficiency and Maternal Health." Unpublished draft. The World Bank, Washington, D.C.

Argüello, S. 1988. "Etología de la medicina tradicional ecuatoriana: el caso de mal aire." En L. McKee y S. Argüello, eds., *Nuevas Investigaciones antropológicas ecuatorianas.* Quito: Editorial Abya-Yala.

Balladelli, P. with J. M. Colcha. 1996. *Entre lo Mágico y lo Natural: la Medicina Indígena, Testimonios de Pesillo.* (3rd ed.) Quito: Ediciones Abya-Yala.

Barker, D. J. P. 1992. *Fetal and Infant Origins of Adult Disease.* London: British Medical Journal Publishing Group.

———. 1994. "Mothers, Babies, and Disease in Later Life." London: British Medical Journal Publishing Group.

Barrera, A. 1990. "The Role of Maternal Schooling and Its Interactions with Public Health Programs in Child Health Production." *Journal of Development Economics* 32.

Becker, G. 1981. *A Treatise on the Family.* Cambridge: Harvard University Press.

Behrman, J. R., and A. B. Deolalikar. 1988. "Health and Nutrition." In H. Chenery and T. N. Srinivasan, eds., *Handbook of Development Economics.* Amsterdam: Elsever Science Publishers.

Berti, Peter R., William R. Leonard, and Wilma J. Berti. 1998. "Stunting in an Andean Community: Prevalence and Etiology." *American Journal of Human Biology* 10(2): 229–40.

Bianchi, César. 1993. "Hombre y Mujer en la Sociedad Shuar." Quito: Ediciones Abya-Yala.

Branca, F., and M. Ferrari. 2002. "Impact of Micronutrient Deficiencies on Growth: The Stunting Syndrome." *Annals of Nutrition & Metabolism* 46:8–17.

Burgard, Sarah. 2004. "Race and Pregnancy-related Care in Brazil and South Africa." *Social Science and Medicine* 59:1127–1146.

Bustos, P., H. Amigo, S. R. Munoz, and R. Martorell. 2001. "Growth in Indigenous and Non-indigenous Chilean Schoolchildren from 3 Poverty Strata." *American Journal of Public Health* 91(10):1645–9.

Carroll, T. F., ed. 2002. "Construyendo Capacidades Colectivas: Fortalecimiento organizativo de las federaciones campesinas-indígenas en la Sierra ecuatoriana." Quito: Soka University of America, World Bank Group Danish Trust Fund, PRODEPINE, The World Bank Group Fondo Sociedad Civil, Oxfam America, Heifer Internacional.

Castillo, C., E. Atalah, J. Riumallo, and R. Castro. 1996. "Breast-feeding and the Nutritional Status of Nursing Children in Chile. *Bulletin of the Pan American Health Organization* 30(2):125–133.

Chaning-Pearce, S. M., and L. Solomon. 1986. "A Longitudinal Study of Height and Weight in Black and White Johannesburg Children." *South African Medical Journal* 70:743–746.

Chaparro, C. M., L. M. Neufeld, G. Tena Alavez, R. Eguia-Líz Cedillo, and K. G. Dewey. 2006, "Effect of Timing of Umbilical Cord Clamping on Iron Status in Mexican Infants: A Randomised Controlled Trial." *The Lancet* 367(9527):1997–2004.

Chirapaq website: http://www.chirapaq.org.pe/htm/segurset.htm.

Clegg, E. J., I. G. Pawson, E. H. Ashton, and R. M. Finn. 1972. "The Growth of Children at Different Altitudes in Ethiopia." *Philos Trans Soc Land* 264:403–37.

Coady, D., Margaret Grosh, and John Hoddinott. 2003. "Targeting outcomes *redux*." Washington, D.C.: International Food Policy Research Institute.

Coady, N. D., and J. Maluccio. 2004. IADB working paper RE2—0404—012012.

Cook, J. D., E. Boy, C. Flowers, and Daroca. 2005. "The Influence of High-altitude Living on Body Iron." *Blood* 106(4):1441–1446.

De Meer, K., H. S. A. Heymans, and W. G. Zijlstra. 1995. "Physical Adaptation of Children to Life at High Altitude." *European Journal of Pediatrics* 154:263–72.

De Onis, M., C. G. Victora, C. Garza, E. A. Frongillo Jr., and T. J. Cole. 2001. "A New International Growth Reference for Young Children." In P. Dasgupta and R. Hauspie, eds., *Perspectives in Human Growth, Development and Maturation*. Dordrecht, The Netherlands: Kluwer Academic Publishers.

De Onis, M., C. Garza, and J.-P. Habicht. 2006. "Time for a New Growth Reference." *PEDIATRICS* 100(5).

Del Pozo, J. 2003. "Ñukanchik Mishki Mikuna: La seguridad alimentaria en los pueblos andinos. El caso de la Asociación Agroartesanal 'Transito Amaguana.'" Quito: Editorial Abya Yala.

Del Rosso, Joy Miller. 1999. "School Feeding Programs: Improving Effectiveness and Increasing the Benefit to Education, A Guide for Program Managers." The Partnership for Child Development. http://www.schoolsandhealth.org/download%20docs/School%20Feeding%20Del%20Rosso%20June%2099.pdf.

Dewey, Kathryn. 2006. "Window of Opportunity for Impacting Child Nutritional Status." February Presentation, Program in International and Community Nutrition, University of California, Davis.

DHS data for Nicaragua accessed at http://www.measuredhs.com/pubs/pub_details.cfm? ID=373&SrvyTp=DHS&ctry_id=54.

Doak, C. 2002. "Large-scale Interventions and Programs Addressing Nutrition-Related Chronic Diseases and Obesity: Examples from 14 Countries." *Public Health Nutrition* 5(1A):253–61.

Dolan, C., and F. J. Levinson. 2000. "Will We Ever Get Back?" Report prepared for the UNICEF-World Bank Nutrition Assessment Project. The World Bank, Washington, D.C.

Eggleston, E. 1999. "Determinants of Unintended Pregnancy among Women in Ecuador." *International Family Planning Perspectives* 25(1): 27–33.

El Comercio. 2006a. "La atención de Maternidad Gratuita está en serio peligro." March, 24:20.

———. 2006b. "Indígenas aprenden sobre el parto limpio." April, 3:19.

ENDEMAIN (Encuesta Demográfica y de Salud Materna e Infantil). 2004. Informe Preliminar.

Escobar Konanz, M. 1990. *La Frontera Imprecisa: lo Natural y lo Sagrado en el Norte de Esmeraldas.* Quito: Centro cultural Afro-Ecuatoriano.

Escobar Quiñonez, R. (nd). *Memoria Viva: Costumbres y Tradiciones Esmeraldeñas.* Taller de Arte y Cultura Negra Ecuatoriana Ël Canoita.

Estrella, E. 1978. *Medicina Aborigen.* Quito: Editorial Época.

———. 1991. "Función maternal y sexualidad: un estudio de una población campesina en la provincia de Pichincha." *Hombre y Ambiente* 5(18):5–130.

Eveleth, P. B., and J. M. Tanner. 1976. *Worldwide Variation in Human Growth.* Cambridge: Cambridge University Press.

———. 1990. *Worldwide Variation in Human Growth.* Second Edition. Cambridge: Cambridge University Press.

FAO (Food and Agriculture Organization). Focus: The Developing World's New Burden: Obesity. http://www.fao.org/FOCUS/E/obesity/obes2.htm.

———. 2001. "Perfil Nutricional de Ecuador, Lineamentos de Politica sobre Seguridad Alimentaria y Nutricion." Octubre.

FAO SOFS. 2004. As cited in IFPRI. "The Economic Rationale for Improving Nutrition." PowerPoint Presentation, May, 2006.

Fiedler, J. 2003. "A Cost Analysis of the Honduras Community-based, Integrated Child Care Program." Health, Nutrition and Population (HNP) Discussion Paper. The World Bank, Washington, D.C.

Finerman, R. D. 1983. "Experience and Expectation: Conflict and Change in Traditional Family Health Care among the Quechua of Saraguro." *Social Science and Medicine* 17(17):1291–8.

———. 1984. "A Matter of Life and Death: Health Care Changes in an Andean Community." *Social Science and Medicine* 18(4):329–34.

———. 1991. "Inside Out: Women's World View and Family Health in an Ecuadorian Indian Community." *Social Science and Medicine* 25(10):1157–62.

———. "The Burden of Responsibility: Duty, Depression, and Nervios in Andean Ecuador." *Health Care Women International* 10(2–3):141–57.

Finerman, R. D., and R. Sackett. 2003. "Using Home Gardens to Decipher Health and Healing in the Andes." *Medical Anthropology Quarterly* 17(4):459–82.

Flores, R. 2006. Interview. March 24.

Forsdal, A. 1977. "Are Poor Living Conditions in Childhood and Adolescence an Important Risk Factor for Arteriosclerotic Heart Disease?" *British Journal of Preventive and Social Medicine* 31(1):91–95.

Foster, G. M. 1976. "Disease Etiologies in Non-western Medical Systems." *American Anthropologist* 78(4):773–82.

———. 1978. *Hippocrates' Latin American Legacy: Humoral Medicine in the New World.* New York: Gordan & Breach Science Publications.

Freire, W. (nd). "Los patrones de consumo y el prestigio de los alimentos." *Identidad* 1:16–18.

———. 1989. "Hemoglobin as a Predictor of Response to Iron Therapy and its Use in Screening and Prevalence Estimates." *American Journal of Clinical Nutrition* 50: 1442–9.

Freire, W., H. Dirren, J. O. Mora, P. Arenales, E. Granda, J. Breilh, A. Campaña, R. Paéz, L. Darquea, and E. Molina. 1988. "Diagnóstico de la situación alimentaria y nutricional y de salud de la población ecuatoriana menor de cinco años -DANS-1986." Consejo Nacional del Desarrollo, Ministerio de Salud Publica, Quito.

Freire, Wilma A. (editor). 2005. "Nutrition and an Active Life: From Knowledge to Action. Washington, D.C." Pan-American Health Organization.

Frisancho, A. R., and P. T. Baker. 1970. "Altitude and Growth: A Study of the Patterns of Physical Growth of a High Altitude Quechua Population." *American Journal of Physical Anthropology* 32:279–92.

Frongillo, E. A., and K. M. P. Hanson. 1995. "Determinants of Variability among Nations in Child Ggrowth." *Annals of Human Biology* 22:395–41.

Garrett, James L., and Marie T. Ruel. "Stunted Child-Overweight Mother Pairs: An Emerging Policy Concern." Discussion Paper Briefs, International Food Policy Research Institute (IFRPRI). Discussion Paper 148.

Glewwe, Paul, and Hanan Jacoby. 1994. "Student Achievement and Schooling Choice in Low Income Countries: Evidence from Ghana." *Journal of Human Resources* 29(3):843–864.

Glick, Peter, Alessandra Marini, and David E. Sahn. 2006 (forthcoming). "Estimating the Consequences of Unintended Fertility for Child Health and Education in Romania: An Analysis Using Twins Data." *Oxford Bulletin of Economics and Statistics.*

Goicolea, I. 2001. "Exploring Women's Needs in an Amazonian Region of Ecuador. *Reproductive Health Matters* 9(17):193–202.

Gordillo, Amparo. 2003. "Costos, Cobertura y Financiamiento del Programa PANN 2000, Ecuador 2000–2003." Programa de Políticas Publicas y Sistemas de Salud, Organización Panamericana de la Salud.

Greska, L. P. 1986a. "Chest Morphology of Young Bolivia High-altitude Residents of European Ancestry." *Human Biology* 58:427–443.

———. 1986b. "Growth Patterns of Europeans and Amerindian High-Altitude Natives." *Current Anthropology* 27(1):72–4.

Griffiths, M., and J. McGuire. 2004. "A New Dimension for Health Reform: Atención Integral a la Ninez en la Comunidad in Honduras." Draft monograph

Guerrón, C. 2000. *El Color de la Panela.* Quito: Centro Cultural Afroecuatoriano.

Guissani, Dino, A. P. Seamus Phillips, Syd Anstee, and David J. P. Barker. 2001. "Effects of Altitude *versus* Economic Status on Birth Weight and Body Shape at Birth." *Pediatric Research* 49(4).

Gujurat Health: www.gujhealth.gov.i (Health and Family Welfare Dept., "Review Meet-ings" and "Grading Primary Health Centers").

Haas, J. D., E. F. Frongillo, C. Stepcik, J. Beard, and L. Hurtado. 1980. "Altitude, Ethnic, and Sex Differences in Birthweight and Length in Bolivia." *Human Biology* 52:459–477.

Haas, J. D., G. Moreno-Black, E. A. Frongillo, J. Pabo, G. Pareja, J. Ybarnegaray, and L. Hurtado. 1982. "Altitude and Infant Growth in Bolivia: A Longitudinal Study." *American Journal of Physical Anthropology* 59:251–62.

Habicht, J.-P., R. Martorell, C. Yarbrough, R. M. Malina, and R.E. Klein. 1974. "Height and Weight Standards for Preschool Children. How Relevant Are Ethnic Differences in Growth Potential." *Lancet* 6:611–614.

Habicht, J.-P., C. Yarbrough, A. Lechtig, and R. E. Klein. 1973. "Relationship of Birth Weight, in Maternal Nutrition and Infant Mortality." *Nutr. Repr. Int.* 7:533–46.

Haddad, L., H. Alderman, S. Appleton, L. Song, and Y. Yones. 2002. "Reducing Child Undernutrition: How Far Does Income Growth Take Us?" FCND Discussion Paper No. 137, International Food Policy Research Institute, Washington, D.C.

Hall, Gillette, and Harry Anthony Patrinos. 2005. "Indigenous Peoples, Poverty and Human Development in Latin America: 1994–2004." The World Bank, Washington, D.C.

Hamilton, S. 1998. *The Two-Headed Household: Gender and Rural Development in the Ecuadorian Andes.* Pittsburgh: University of Pittsburg Press.

Harari, R., R. Ghersi, N. Comi, M. Ganguera, G. Lecota, and J. F. Harare. 2000. *Trabajo y Salud en el Ecuador: Antecedentes, Experiencias y Perspectivas.* Quito: Ediciones Abya Yala.

Harner, M. J. 1994. *Shuar: Pueblo de las Cascadas Sagradas.* Quito: Ediciones Abya-Yala.

Harris, Nancy S., Patricia B. Crawford, Yeshe Yangzom, Lobsang Pinzo, Palden Gyaltsen, and Mark Hudes. 2001. "Nutritional and Health Status of Tibetan Children Living at High Altitudes." *New England Journal of Medicine* 344(5): 341–347.

Heaver, R., and Y. Kachondam. 2002. "Thailand's National Nutrition Program: Lessons in Management and Capacity Building." Health, Nutrition and Population Discussion Paper, The World Bank, Washington, D.C.

Hentschel, J., and W. F. Waters. 1996. "Rural Poverty in Ecuador—A Qualitative Assess-ment." Policy Research Working Paper 1576, Latin America and the Caribbean Coun-try Department III Country Operations Division 1, The World Bank, Washington, D.C.

Herrera, G., M. C. Carrillo, and A. Torres, eds. 2005. *La Migración Ecuatoriana: Transna-cionalismo, Redes e Identidades.* Quito: FLACSO.

Herrera, J. 1978. *La familia en la sociedad afro-americana.* Esmeraldas, Ecuador: Secretari-ado de Promoción Humana, Vicariato de Esmeraldas.

Herrera, M. 2000. "Breast Feeding and Milk Insufficiency in Esmeraldas City, Ecuador: A Biocultural Perspective." Research in Public Health Technical Papers, Pan-American Health Organization, Washington, D.C.

Hess, E. 1994. "Enfermedad y moralidad en los Andes Ecuatorianos." In P. Warren, C. Hess, E. Ferraro, and L. Agassiz, (eds.), *Salud y Antropología. Hombre y Ambiente* No. 29. Quito: Ediciones Abya-Yala.

Hinrichsen, D. 1999. "Taking Health to the High Sierra. Millennium Trailblazers 4: Jambi Huasi." *People Planet* 8:21–22.

———. 2006. "Trabajo desde adentro y desde afuera." United Nations Population Fund. http://www.unfpa.org/news/news.cfm?ID=742&Language=2. Accessed April 3, 2006.

HKI Nutrition Bulletin: Nepal. 2004. 2(1).

HNP. 2002. "Food Policy Options: Preventing and Controlling Nutrition Related Non-Communicable Diseases." Discussion paper. WHO/World Bank. November.

Horton, Susan. 1986. "Child Nutrition and Family Size in the Philippines." *Journal of Development Economics* 23(1):161–76.

Horwitz, Abraham. 1987. "Comparative Public Health: Costa Rica, Cuba, and Chile." *Food and Nutrition Bulletin* 9(3), September. The United Nations University Press.

Huijbers, P. M. J. F, J. L. M. Hendriks, W. J. M. Gerver, P. J. de Jong, and K de Meer. 1996. "Nutritional Status and Mortality of Highland Children in Nepal: Impact of Socio-cultural Factors." *American Journal of Physical Anthropology* 101:137–144.

IADB (Inter-American Development Bank). 2006. "Operational Policy on Indigenous Peoples." February. http://www.iadb.org/sds/doc/IND-PGN2386E.pdf.

IDPAS website. http://www.idpas.org/pdf/1975AdvancesinIronFortificationPPT.pdf.

IESS (Instituto Ecuatoriano de Seguridad Social). 2006. Estadísticas IESS. www.iess.gov.ed. Accessed March 31, 2006.

IFPRI. 2002. "Sistema de evaluación de la fase piloto de la Red de Protección Social de Nicaragua: Evaluación de focalización." Report submitted to the Red de Protección Social. Washington, D.C.

Instituto de Ciencia y tecnología/Ministerio de Salud Publica. 1999. "La deficiencia de Vitamina A en los niños Ecuatoriano." *Boletin Informativo del ITC N*, 2. Quito, Mayo.

James, Philip, Rachel Leach, Eleni Kalamara, and Maryam Shayeghi. 2001. "The Worldwide Obesity Epidemic." *Obesity Research* 9:S228-S233. http://www.obesityresearch.org/cgi/content/full/9/suppl_4/S228.

Kavishe, F. P. 1993. "Nutrition Relevant Actions in Tanzania." Paper presented to the UN Subcommittee on Nutrition.

Keller, W. 1983. "Choice of Indicators of Nutritional Status." In B. Schurch, ed., *Evaluation of Nutrition Education in Third World Communities*. Nestle' Foundation Publication Series. Bern: Hans Huber Publishers.

Kolenikov, S., and G. Angeles. 2004. "Construction of the SES Indices from Discrete Data by PCA." MEASURE Evaluation Working Paper Draft. Atlanta: MEASURE.

Kroeger, A. 1982a. "South American Indians between Traditional and Modern Health Services in Rural Ecuador." *Bulletin of the Pan-American Health Organization* 16(3):242–54.

———. 1982b. "Participatory Evaluation of Primary Health Care Programmes: An Experience with Four Indian Populations in Ecuador." *Tropical Doctor* 12(1):38–43.

Kroeger, A., and H. P. Franken. 1981. "The Educational Value of Participatory Evaluation of Primary Health Care Programmes: An Experience with Four Indigenous Populations in Ecuador." *Social Science and Medicine* 15(4):535–39.

Kroeger, A., and E. Ilechkova. 1983. *Salud y Alimentación Shuar*. Quito: Mundo Shuar.

Kyle, D. 2000. *Transnational Peasants: Migrations, Networks, and Ethnicity in Andean Ecuador*. Baltimore and London: The Johns Hopkins University Press.

Larrea, C., P. Montalvo, and A. M. Ricaurte. 2004. "Child Malnutrition, Social Development and Health Services in the Andean Region." Second Progress Report, FLACSO, Ecuador. January.

———. 2005. "Child Malnutrition, Social Development and Health Services in the Andean Region." FLACSO, Ecuador, April.

Lavy, V., J. Strauss, D. Thomas, and P. de Vreyer. 1996. "Quality of Health Care, Survival and Health Outcomes in Ghana." *Journal of Health Economics* 15(3):333–57.

Lefeber, Yvonne, and Henk W. A. Voorhoeve. 1998. *Indigenous Customs in Childbirth and Child Care.* Van Gorcum.

Leonard, W. R., K. M. DeWalt, J. P. Stansbury, and M. K. McCaston. 2003. "Influence of Dietary Quality on the Growth of Highland and Coastal Ecuadorian Children." *American Journal of Human Biology* 12(6):825–37.

Leonard, W. R., T. L. Leatherman, J. W. Carey, and R. B. Thomas. 1990. "Contributions of Nutrition Versus Hypoxia to Growth in Rural Andean Populations." *American Journal of Human Biology* 2:613–26.

Lutter, C. "Un ejemplo de un Nuevo modelo para la ayuda económica alimentaria." PANN, PAHO. Feb. 2001. http://www.paho.org/Spanish/HPP/HPN/PANN2000español.pdf.

Maradiaga, A., M. Griffiths, and I. Nunez. 1997. "Pacticas mejoradas de alimentacion." Tegucigalpa: Ministerio de Salud and BASICS.

Marini, Alessandra, and Michele Gragnolati. 2006. "Nonlinear Effects of Altitude on Child Growth in Peru: A Multilevel Analysis." World Bank Policy Research Working Paper No. 3823. Washington, D.C.

———. 2003. "Malnutrition and Poverty in Guatemala." World Bank Policy Research Working Paper No. 2967. Washington, D.C.

Marquez, Patricio, and Willy deGeyndt. 2003. "Mexico: Reaching the Poor with Basic Health Services." World Bank. En Breve No. 20, March.

Martínez, L. 2003. "Endogenous Peasant Responses to Structural Adjustment: Ecuador in Comparative Andean Perspective." In L. L. North and J. D. Cameron, eds., *Rural Progress, Rural Decay.* Bloomfield, CT: Kumarian.

Martorell, R. 1985. "Child Growth Retardation: A Discussion of Its Causes and Its Relationships to Health." In K. Blaxter and J. C. Tanner, eds., *Nutritional Adaptation in Man.* London: John Libbey.

———. 2001. "Obesity." 2020 Focus No. 05-Brief 07. February. http://www.ifpri.org/2020/focus/focus05/focus05%5F07.asp.

Martorell, R., and J.-P. Habicht. 1986. "Growth in Early Childhood in Developing Countries. In F. Falkner and J. M. Tanner, eds., *Human Growth: A Comprehensive Treatise,* Volume 3. New York: Plenum Press.

Martorell, R., J. Leslie, and P. R. Moock. 1984. "Characteristics and Determinants of Child Nutritional Status in Nepal." *American Journal of Clinical Nutrition* 39:74–86.

Martorell, R., and N. S. Scrimshaw. 1995. "The Effects of Improved Nutrition in Early Childhood." The Institute of Nutrition of Central America and Panamá (INCAP). Follow-up study, *Journal of Nutrition* S125: 4.

Mason, Jhon B., Philip Musgrove, and Jean-Pierre Habicht. 2003. "At Least One Third of Poor Countries' Disease Burden is Due to Malnutrition." Working Paper No. 1, Disease Control Priorities Project, Fogarty International Center, National Institutes of Health, Bethesda, Maryland.

McKee, L. 1987. "Controles tradicionales de la reproducción en la sierra ecuatoriana: efectos en la estructura demográfica." *Hombre y Ambiente* 1(1):131–40.

———. 1988. "Tratamiento etnomédico de las enfermedades diarreicas de los niños de la Sierra del Ecuador." En L. McKee y S. Argüello, (eds.), *Nuevas Investigaciones Antropológicas Ecuatorianas.* Quito: Editorial Abya-Yala.

MEC-PAE, PNUD, UNESCO (Ministerio de Educación y Cultura-Programa de Alimentación Escolar, Programa de las Naciones Unidas para el Desarrollo, United

Nations Educational, Scientific and Cultural Organization). 2006. "Línea de base del Programa de alimentación Escolar." May.

Micronutrient Initiative. 2002. "Report on Wheat Flour Fortification in Latin America." (Internal document). Ottawa.

———. 2004. *Fortification Handbook.* Ottawa.

Ministerio de Salud Pública. www.msp.gov.ec.

Ministerio de Salud Pública—PANN 2000. "Manual Operativo PANN 2000."

Ministerio de Salud Pública—Organización Panamericana de la Salud – PANN 2000. "Evaluación de impacto Mi papilla." 2005.

Moock, Peter R., and Joanne Leslie. 1986. "Childhood Malnutrition and Schooling in the Terai Region of Nepal." *Journal of Development Economics* 20:33–52.

Morales, Rolando, Ana Maria Aguilar, and Alvaro Calzadilla. 2005. "Undernutrition in Bolivia: Geography and Culture Matter." Working Paper #R-492. Latin American Research Network, Research Network, Inter-American Development Bank, Washington, D.C.

Mosley, W. H., and L. Chen. 1984. "An Analytical Framework for the Study of Child Survival in Developing Countries." In W. H. Mosley and L. C. Chen, eds., *Child Survival: Strategies for Research, Supplement to Population and Development Review 10.*

MSP. 1995. "Programa Integrado para el Control de las Principales Deficiencias de Micronutrientes en el Ecuador." Quito. October.

MSP/INEC (Ministerio de Salud Pública/Instituto Nacional de Estadística y Censo). 2005. "Indicadores Básicos de Salud. Ecuador 2005." Quito: MPS/INEC.

Mueller, W. 1986. "The Genetics of Size and Shape in Children and Adults." In F. Falkner and J. M. Tanner, *Human Growth: A Comprehensive Treatise,* Volume 3. New York: Plenum Press.

Mueller, W. H., V. N. Schull, W. J. Schull, P. Soto, and F. Rothhammer. 1978. "A Multinational Andean Genetic and Health Program: Growth and Development in an Hypoxic Environment." *Annals of Human Biology* 5(4):329–52.

Muñoz Bernard, C. 1999. "Enfermedad, Daño e Ideología." Quito: Ediciones Abya-Yala.

Myers, R. G. 1994. "Childrearing Practices in Latin America: Summary of the Workshop Results." http://www.ecdgroup.com/download/cc115ccl.pdf. Retrieved April 3, 2006.

Nalubola, R., and P. Nestel. 2000. "Manual for Wheat Flour Fortification with Iron Part 3, Analytical Methods for Monitoring Wheat Flour Fortification with Iron." The MOST Project, Washington, D.C.

Naranjo, M. (nd). *La Cultura Popular en el Ecuador: Tomo IV: Esmeraldas.* Quito: Centro Interamericano de Artesanías y Artes Populares (CIDAP).

———. 1984. *La Cultura Popular en el Ecuador: Tomo V: Imbabura.* Quito: Centro Interamericano de Artesanías y Artes Populares (CIDAP).

NARI: High Altitude Highlands Livestock http://www.nari.org.pg/research/hahp/-livestock.htm.

Naula, S. 2006. Personal interview. Local indigenous leader (female) and key informant in Chimborazo Province, Ecuador. February 1.

Nestel, P., R. Nalubola, and others. 2002. "Quality Assurance as Applied to Micronutrient Fortification." ILSI, Washington, D.C.

Novotny, R. 1986. "Preschool Child Feeding, Health and Nutritional Status in Highland Ecuador." Ph.D. Dissertation, Cornell University.

———. 1987. "Preschool Child Feeding, Health and Nutritional Status in Gualaceo, Ecuador." *Archivos Latinoamericanos de Nutrición* 37(3):417–33.

———. 1988. "Alimentación, salud y estado nutricional del niño preescolar en la Sierra Ecuatoriana." En L. McKee y S. Argüello, (eds.), *Nuevas Investigaciones Antropológicas Ecuatorianas*. Quito: Editorial Abya-Yala.

Nugent, Rachel. 2005. "Obesity-related Diseases Creep Up on Developing Countries." Population Reference Bureau.

Obert, P., N. Fellmann, and G. Falgairette. 1994. "The Importance of Socioeconomic and Nutritional Conditions Rather than Altitude on the Physical Growth of Prepubertal Andean Highland Boys." *Annals of Human Biology* 21:145–54.

Oduber, Daniel. 1987. "The Costa Rican Experience in Improving Nutrition and Health Care." *Food and Nutrition Bulletin* 9(3), September. The United Nations University Press.

Ordoñez J., P. Stupp, G. Angeles, A. Valle, D. Williams, R. Monteigh, and M. Goodwin. 2005. "Encuesta Nacional de Demografía y Salud Materna Infantil – 2004 ENDEMAIN." Informe Final." CEPAR, Centers for Disease Control, MEASURE Evaluation. Quito, Ecuador.

Ordóñez, S. 2005. "Nutritional and Health Behavior of the Indigenous Pregnant Women in the Community of Tunshi-San Nicolas, Chimborazo Province, Ecuador." *Benson Institute.* http://patriot.lib.byu.edu/u?/Benson,4182. Retrieved March 14, 2006.

Ortega, F. 1988. "El contexto cultural de los alimentos." *Hombre y Ambiente* 2(5):103–16).

PAHO (Pan-American Health Organization). 2003. "Flour Fortification with Iron, Folic Acid and Vitamin B12 in the Americas." Background document for regional meeting.

PAHO Newsletter: Indigenous People. May 2004. http://www.paho.org/English/AD/THS /OS/IndigN-vle2_ENG.htm.

PAHO Country Profiles – Bolivia. http://www.paho.org/English/DD/AIS/cp_068.htm.

Partnership for Child Development (PCD). "School Health and Nutrition: A Situation Analysis." http://www.schoolsandhealth.org/download%20docs/English%20Situation%20 Analysis%20June%201999.pdf.

Pawson, I. G. 1977. "Growth Characteristics of Populations of Tibetan Origin in Nepal." *American Journal of Physical Anthropology* 47(3):473–82.

Pawson, Ivan G., Luis Huicho, Manuel Muro, and Alberto Pacheco. 2001. "Growth of Children in Two Economically Diverse Peruvian High-altitude Communities." *American Journal of Physical Anthropology* 13(3):323–40.

Paxson, Christina, and Norbert Schady. 2007 (forthcoming). "Cognitive Development among Young Children in Ecuador: The Roles of Wealth, Health, and Parenting." *Journal of Human Resources* (42):1.

Pebley, A. R., E. Hurtado, and N. Goldman. 1999. "Beliefs about Children's Illness Among Rural Guatemalan Women." *Journal of Biosocial Sciences* 31:195–219.

Pigott, J., and K. Kolasa. 1983. "Infant Feeding Practices and Beliefs in One Community in the Sierra of Rural Ecuador: A Prevalence Study." *Archivos Latinoamericanos de Nutrición* 33(1):126–38.

Platin, A. 2003. "Knowledge, Attitudes & Practices of Quichua Women from Quiturco, Morochos & San Martin Communities in Relation to Social, Economical and Health Development in the High Rural Andes of Imbabura, Ecuador." B.S. thesis, Universidad San Francisco de Quito.

Tufts University. 2001. "Reducción de la desnutrición crónica en el Perú: Propuesta para una estrategia Nacional." Medford, MA.

UN (United Nations). *Human Development Report, 2005.* http://hdr.undp.org/reports/global/2002/en/indicator/cty_f_NIC.html.

UNICEF. 1993. "We Will Never Go Back. Social Mobilisation in the Child Survival and Development Programme in the United Republic of Tanzania."

———. 1999. "Mid-term review of Government of Tanzania/UNICEF Country Programme, 1997–2001."

———. 2004. *State of the World's Children.* New York.

———. 2005. *Estado Mundial de la Infancia 2006: Excluidos e Invisibles.* New York.

United Nations Subcommittee on Nutrition. 2004. Fifth Report on the World Nutrition Situation, Annex 6: Overweight and Obesity.

Uzendoski, M. 2005. *The Napo Runa of Amazonian Ecuador.* Urbana and Chicago: University of Illinois Press.

Van Roekel, K., B. Plowman, M. Griffiths, V. De Alvarado, J. Matute, and M. Calderon. 2002. BASICS II. "Midterm Evaluation of the AIN Program in Honduras, 2002." Arlington, VA: BASICS.

Victora, C. G., J. P. Vaughan, B. R. Kirkwood, J. C. Martines, and L. B. Barcelos. 1986. "Risk Factors for Malnutrition in Brazilian Children: The Role of Social and Environmental Variables." *Bulletin of the World Health Organization* 64(2):299–309.

Victora, C. G., J. P. Vaughan, J. C. Martines, and L. B. Barcelos. 1984. "Is Prolonged Breastfeeding Associated with Malnutrition?" *American Journal of Clinical Nutrition* 39:307–314.

Vincent, David, Marco Moncada, and Fidel Ordonez. 2004. "Private and Public Determinants of Child Nutrition in Nicaragua and the Western regions of Honduras." Latin American Research Network Project, Inter-American Development Bank, Washington, D.C., March.

Vitzthum, V. J. 2001. "The Home Team Advantage: Reproduction in Women Indigenous to High Altitude." *Journal of Experimental Biology* 204:3141–3150.

Waterlow, J. R., W. Buzina, W. Keller, J. Lane, M. Nichaman, and J. Tanner. 1977. "The Presentation and Use of Height and Weight Data for Comparing the Nutritional Status of Groups of Children under the Age of 10 Years." *Bulletin of the World Health Organization* 55(4):489–98.

Waters, W. F. 1997. "The Road of Many Returns: Rural Bases of the Informal Urban Economy." *Latin American Perspectives* 24(3):52–66.

———. 2006. "Salud, transición y globalización: la experiencia del Ecuador." In X. Sosa-Buchholz and W. F. Waters, eds., *Estudios Ecuatorianos: Un Aporte a la Discusión.* Quito: Abya Yala/FLACSO/Sección de Estudios Ecuatorianos LASA.

Waters, W. F., and F. H. Buttel. 1987. "Differenciación sin descampesinización: acceso a la tierra y persistencia del campesinado andino ecuatoriano." *Estudios Rurales Latinoamericanos* (Bogotá, Colombia) 10(3):355–78.

Weber J. T., E. D. Mintz, R. Canizares, A. Semiglia, I. Gomez, R. Sempertegui, A. Davila, K. D. Greene, N. D. Puhr, D. N. Cameron, et al. 1994. "Epidemic Cholera in Ecuador: Multidrug-resistance and Transmission by Water and Seafood." *Epidemiology and Infection* 112(1):1–11.

Weigel, M. M., and N. P. Castro. 2001. "Adquisición de alimentos, prácticas alimentarias y estado nutricional de mujeres minoritarias de ascendencia africana que viven en la región tropical de América del Sur." Pan-American Health Organization, Washington, D.C.

Weismantel, M. J. 1988. *Food, Gender, and Poverty in the Ecuadorian Andes.* Philadelphia: University of Pennsylvania Press.

WFP http://www.wfp.org/food_aid/school_feeding/LearnMore_Publications.asp?section =12&sub_section=3.

Whitten, N. 1997 [1965]. *Los Negros de San Lorenzo: Clase, Parentesco y Poder en un Pueblo Ecuatoriano.* Quito: Centro Cultural Afroecuatoriano.

———. 1992. *La cultura afro-latinoamericana del Ecuador y Colombia.* Quito: Centro Cultural Afro-Ecuatoriano.

Whitten, S., and N. E. Whitten. 1985. *Art, Knowledge, and Health: Development and Assessment of a Collaborative, Auto-financed Organization in Eastern Ecuador.* Cambridge, MA: Cultural Survival, Inc.

Wiecha J. L., K. E. Peterson, D. S. Ludwig, J. Kim, A. Sobol, and S. L. Gortmaker. 2006. "When Children Eat What They Watch." *Archives of Pediatrics and Adolescent Medicine* 160(April):436–42.

Wood, Charles H., and Jose Alberto Magno De Carvalho. 1988. "The Demography of Inequality in Brazil." London: Cambridge University Press.

Wood, Charles H., and Peggy A. Lovell. 1992. "Racial Inequality and Child Mortality in Brazil." *Social Forces* 70(3):703–724.

World Bank. 1993. *World Development Report 1993: Investing in Health.* New York: Oxford University Press for the World Bank.

———. 1997a. "Honduras Improving Access, Efficiency and Quality of Care in the Health Sector." Report no. 17008-HO. Washington, D.C.

———. 1997b. *World Development Indicators.* Washington, D.C.

———. 2002. *Poverty and Nutrition in Bolivia.* A World Bank Country Study, Washington, D.C.

World Bank website on Indigenous Peoples, Poverty and Human Development in Latin America: 1994–2004. http://web.worldbank.org/WBSITE/EXTERNAL/COUNTRIES/ LACEXT/0,,contentMDK:20505836~menuPK:258559~pagePK:146736~piPK:226340 ~theSitePK:258554,00.html.

World Health Organization. 1979. *Measurement of Nutritional Impact.* Geneva.

———. 1983. *Measuring Change in Nutritional Status.* Geneva.

World Health Organization Working Group. 1986. "Use and Interpretation of Anthropometric Indicators of Nutritional Status." *Bulletin of the World Health Organization* 64:924–41.

World Health Organization Working Group on Infant Growth. 1995. "An Evaluation of Infant Growth: The Use and Interpretation of Anthropometry in Infants." *Bulletin of the World Health Organization* 73(2):165–74.

World Health Organization, United Nations Children Fund, and International Council for Control of Iodine Deficiency Disorders. 1993. "Global Prevalence of Iodine Deficiency Disorders." Micronutrient Deficiency Information System Working Paper #1. July.

Zamosc, L. 2003. "Agrarian Protest and the Indian Movement in the Ecuadorian Highlands." In E. D. Langer and E. Muñoz, eds., *Contemporary Indigenous Movements in Latin America.* Wilmington, DE: SR Books.

Zamudio S., T. Droma, K. Y. Norkyel, G. Acharya, J. A. Zamudio, S. N. Nirmeyer, and L. G. Moore. 1993. "Protection from Intrauterine Growth Retardation in Tibetans at High Altitude." *American Journal of Physical Anthropology* 91:215–224.

Eco-Audit

Environmental Benefits Statement

The World Bank is committed to preserving Endangered Forests and natural resources. We print World Bank Working Papers and Country Studies on 100 percent postconsumer recycled paper, processed chlorine free. The World Bank has formally agreed to follow the recommended standards for paper usage set by Green Press Initiative—a nonprofit program supporting publishers in using fiber that is not sourced from Endangered Forests. For more information, visit www.greenpressinitiative.org.

In 2006, the printing of these books on recycled paper saved the following:

Trees*	Solid Waste	Water	Net Greenhouse Gases	Total Energy
203	9,544	73,944	17,498	141 mil.
'40' in height and 6–8" in diameter	Pounds	Gallons	Pounds Co$_2$ Equivalent	BTUs

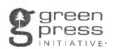